Hospital Strategies for Contracting with Managed Care Plans

Kathryn A. Schroer and Donald A. Penn
William M. Mercer-Meidinger-Hansen, Incorporated

Legal Chapter by Mary Layne Ahern, J.D.
Office of Legal and Regulatory Affairs
American Hospital Association

Edited by Gary J. Rahn
Division of Ambulatory Care
American Hospital Association

American Hospital Publishing, Inc.
a wholly owned subsidiary of the
American Hospital Association

Library of Congress Cataloging-in-Publication Data

Schroer, Kathryn A.
  Hospital strategies for contracting with managed
  care plans.

  "Alternative delivery and financing systems publica-
  tions" — Cover.
  1. Hospitals — Business management.   2. Hospital
care — Contracting out.   3. Managed care plans (Medical
care).   I. Penn, Donald A.   II. Ahern, Mary Layne.
III. Rahn, Gary J.   IV. Title. [DNLM: 1. Financial
Management — methods.   2. Health Maintenance Organizations — organization & administration — United States.
3. Hospital Administration — United States.   4. Insurance,
Health — United States.   WX 157 S381h]
RA971.3.S36   1987   362.1'1'0681   87-18688
ISBN 1-55648-004-0

Catalog no. 067100

©1987 by American Hospital Publishing, Inc.,
a wholly owned subsidiary
of the American Hospital Association

Printed in the U.S.A.

ΛHΛ is a service mark of the American Hospital Association used
under license by American Hospital Publishing, Inc.

Text printed in English Times
2M-8/87-0131
2M-7/87-0217
Sandra L. Weiss, Project Editor
Wayne S. Brown, Managing Editor
Peggy DuMais, Production Coordinator
Marcia Vecchione, Designer
Brian W. Schenk, Books Division Director

Contents

List of Figures

Acknowledgments

The authors gratefully acknowledge the valuable contributions of Joseph H. Rosmann and Gary J. Rahn. They also wish to acknowledge the substantial contribution of Sandra W. Peters in organizing, reviewing, and expediting the development of the manuscript. Our sincere thanks to these individuals.

Foreword

The American Hospital Association convened a task force to look critically at the growth of alternative delivery and financing systems and the hospital industry's response to that growth. The task force developed a conceptual framework for hospital management to use when developing strategies for working with alternative delivery and financing systems. The framework identifies the following areas of the hospital that are affected by these systems and the priority issues that these areas need to consider: executive management, strategic planning, marketing, legal, clinical service delivery, finance, human resources, and administrative services.

One way that hospitals can respond to the challenge of alternative delivery and financing systems is by acting as a contracting provider within a managed care structure. Such managed care plans include health maintenance organizations, competitive medical plans, preferred provider organizations, and provider agreements made directly with employers. This book developed out of the interest expressed by AHA members in definitive information regarding the contracting process. The task force secured the services of A. S. Hansen (now William M. Mercer-Meidinger-Hansen), a benefits consulting firm, to develop a manuscript based on issues identified in the task force's conceptual framework.

Special thanks go to task force members Mary Layne Ahern, John M. Bissinger, Lynn Clayton, Dorothy L. Cobbs, Monica Dreuth,

Eloise Foster, Tom Foster, Diane M. Howard, Heidi Hunter, Steven F. Kukla, Marsha A. Ladenburger, Elizabeth A. Lee, Mark Lundberg, Robert W. McCann, Jo Ellen Mistarz, Henrie Moise, Michael Morrissey, Judy Neiman, Karen Porter, Gary J. Rahn, Sandra L. Weiss, and Gaylen Young.

As the health care industry continues to evolve, managed care initiatives that reduce health care expenditures while ensuring high-quality care and appropriate utilization will become a critical conduit through which patients access hospitals, physicians, and other health care providers. This book assists health care executives in understanding and responding to the environment in which contracting with managed care plans will occur.

Bruce McPherson
Group Vice-President
American Hospital Association

About the Authors

Kathryn A. Schroer, an associate and senior consultant with William M. Mercer-Meidinger-Hansen, manages client assignments in areas relating to health care management nationally. Recent projects for clients include the design, development, and implementation of employer-sponsored, hospital-sponsored, and coalition-sponsored preferred provider programs; feasibility analyses for alternative health management programs; and market surveys for the development of health maintenance organizations and preferred provider organizations. Prior to joining Mercer-Meidinger-Hansen, Ms. Schroer coordinated nationwide alternative delivery system projects for the American Hospital Association. She has published several articles relating to alternative delivery systems and has appeared frequently as a speaker and seminar leader. Ms. Schroer is a graduate of St. Olaf College, Northfield, Minnesota.

Donald A. Penn is currently a partner with the Actuarial, Benefits, and Compensation Consulting Division of Coopers & Lybrand. He was formerly a senior consulting principal in the Deerfield, Illinois, offices of A. S. Hansen, now William M. Mercer-Meidinger-Hansen, where he was responsible for managing client assignments in all areas relating to health care management issues, including developing, analyzing, and recommending the selection of health maintenance organizations, preferred provider organizations, and other health care delivery initiatives. Prior to his involvement with Hansen, Mr. Penn developed and operated one of the country's most cost-effective hospital-based preferred provider organizations and spent more than 15 years with Blue Cross and Blue Shield Plans as an executive responsible for claims administration, data management, and finances. He has served on several regional and national committees relating to health care financing and received his certified professional manager (CM) designation in 1979. Mr. Penn graduated from the University of Northern Colorado in Greeley and did postgraduate work at the University of Michigan in Ann Arbor.

Mary Layne Ahern, J.D., is an assistant general counsel in the American Hospital Association's Office of the General Counsel. In that capacity, she handles a wide variety of issues, including contracting; joint venture arrangements among hospitals, physicians, and other providers of health care services; and tax issues concerning not-for-profit status and parent-subsidiary relationships. In addition, Ms. Ahern chairs AHA's Legal Task Force on Biomedical Ethics and counsels the newly formed AHA Advisory Committee on Biomedical Ethics. She has spoken and written on a number of issues in the field of biomedical ethics. Ms. Ahern was involved in forming AHA's position on the so-called Baby Doe regulations and the subsequent litigation challenging these regulations. She graduated cum laude from Harvard University and received her law degree from DePaul University College of Law in Chicago.

Gary J. Rahn is a member of the professional staff of the American Hospital Association's Division of Ambulatory Care. He is responsible for the initiation, development, and management of activities related to hospital involvement in alternative delivery and financing systems and hospital-sponsored physician group practices. Mr. Rahn was previously on the administrative staff of the University of Chicago Hospitals and Clinics and the systems development staff of the medical center. Mr. Rahn received his master's degree from the University of Chicago Graduate School of Business.

Introduction

Looking to Managed Care

As hospitals strive for continued success in providing health care services, they must become cognizant of the fact that consumers are becoming increasingly concerned about the cost, quality, and appropriateness of care. These purchaser concerns are driving the reshaping of the health care delivery system.

The future of the health care delivery system depends on competitive approaches for organizing, pricing, and delivering high-quality health care services. This trend toward competition is occurring for three principal reasons:

- The excess supply of providers of health care services that exists in many parts of the United States and the resulting reduction in revenue growth
- The desire of government and employers to control further growth in the cost of public health programs and private health insurance
- The social and political commitment to use market forces, rather than regulatory controls, to achieve a better balance between supply and demand factors in the health care economy and to accomplish increased operating efficiencies throughout the system

Competition has fostered the development of systems that integrate financing and delivery in ways other than the traditional fee-for-service systems. Those alternative delivery and financing systems that integrate financing mechanisms, appropriate utilization management, and high-quality service delivery may be considered *managed care plans.* Such systems in effect "manage" care by controlling the selection and utilization of services and provide for appropriate benefits coverage. Thus, health maintenance organizations (HMOs), competitive medical plans (CMPs), preferred provider organizations (PPOs), and direct agreements between employers and providers may be called managed care plans.

This movement toward managed care plans has occurred for several reasons:

- Substantial variation in medical practices and in costs of care among hospitals and physicians treating similar types of patients both locally and regionally have been identified by insurers, employers, and government agencies.
- Health care professionals and organizations have had few economic incentives for providing medical care services efficiently and at reasonable prices.
- Individuals, families, and employees, the consumers of care, are becoming more cost conscious as they assume a greater proportion of the costs of that care.

As the health care delivery system has moved toward managed care, the following practices have emerged:

- Many employers recognize the need to establish more business-like buyer and supplier relationships between themselves and health care providers.
- Health care providers are increasingly willing to accept various external control and audit mechanisms to establish their accountability for both the quality and the cost of their services when these mechanisms are responsibly directed by local community employers and other purchaser groups.
- Many employers have established positive economic incentives in their health care benefits to reward employees for choosing lower cost options.
- Many employers have developed educational programs to assist employees in making better choices in their use of health care services.

- Health care providers have developed processes and programs to achieve the efficiencies required for cost control and to implement marketing mechanisms necessary to meet the impact of competition.
- The insurance industry has responded with the development of new products and services for the marketing and management of managed health care services.

The major objective of all these efforts by private and public payers who are responsible for financing health care benefits programs and by individual consumers is containing health care expenditures and ensuring appropriate utilization and high-quality care. Efforts to fulfill this objective have led employers and government programs, including Medicare and Medicaid, through several developmental stages, which may, in fact, operate simultaneously: first, redesigning their benefits packages to encourage cost-effective use of health care services; then closely monitoring the cost and utilization of services; and finally turning to managed care alternatives. Employers have also moved to assume more of the risk by self-insuring benefits programs and have been increasing their direct links to providers through negotiated direct contracts. These efforts to combine the delivery and financing of health care services have in some instances resulted in decreased hospital admission, decreased average lengths of stay, and stabilized use of ancillary services.

To combat increased competition and their declining utilization, with resulting excess capacity, hospitals are seeking ways to protect or expand their market share. As a result, hospitals have turned to available managed care plans to provide a defined market share.

Health economists predict that more than two-thirds of the American public will be receiving health care services from managed care plans by the mid-1990s. If these predictions become a reality, a majority of the nation's hospitals will provide a significant percentage of their services through managed care contractual arrangements within the next 10 years.

Hospital Strategies for Contracting with Managed Care Plans has been developed to assist health care executives in planning and implementing appropriate competitive strategies for contracting with self-insured employers, PPOs, and HMOs. These strategies, based on realistic and achievable goals, form the foundation of the hospital's bargaining position in contract negotiations.

The increasingly competitive nature of the health care market continues to stimulate the development of new strategies for purchasing health care services. Because of this proliferation of strategies and because each hospital's competitive environment is unique, hospitals will not find one all-encompassing approach that can be universally applied in all competitive contracting situations. Therefore, this book cannot be a handbook for all situations. What the book can do is identify issues, describe approaches, and assess advantages and disadvantages that the hospital chief executive officer and all other involved personnel should be aware of when contracting with employers, PPOs, and HMOs.

A hospital's contracting strategies must be based on a thorough understanding of itself and its market as well as the legal constraints under which it functions. Part I of this book looks at assessing the environment and determining how internal hospital factors and external forces are integrated into the hospital's competitive strategy for working with managed care plans. The chapters in part I help the hospital management team to:

- Examine the hospital's strengths and weaknesses in order to establish the hospital's competitive position
- Determine current service and resource capabilities available to meet market demand and assess associated cost structures
- Understand the administrative systems available to support contracting opportunities
- Assess marketplace trends and future requirements
- Evaluate the effectiveness and scope of competition
- Establish the appropriate level of risk as dictated by the marketplace
- Understand the elements of an effective contract

Part II looks at developing strategies for implementing contracts directly with employers, PPOs, and HMOs. Each type of managed care plan requires the consideration of similar issues and approaches. The chapters in this part of the book are structured to indicate the similarities and highlight the differences among each of these managed care plans. Overall, these chapters help the management team to:

- Determine the advantages and disadvantages of direct employer, PPO, and HMO contracting from a marketplace, financial, and political perspective
- Understand the requirements of each contractual arrangement
- Develop negotiation strategies for contracting with employers, PPOs, and HMOs

Hospitals must realize that managed care plans represent a key force in the future of health care delivery. Because managed care plans provide an opportunity for addressing competitive marketplace forces, hospitals must position themselves to evaluate these plans and to take advantage of appropriate opportunities. Planning for the most advantageous integration into these plans is important to the future viability of hospitals.

Part I

Assessing the Environment

Chapter 1

Evaluating Internal Hospital Factors

Introduction
Hospital Structure and Governance
Mission and Goals
Image
Product Definition
Medical Staff
Technology
Finance
     Pricing and Payer Mix
     Employer Analysis of Costs
     Financial Profiling
     Uncompensated Care
     Data Monitoring Systems
Administrative Staff
Conclusion

Introduction

Current frustrations expressed by many hospital CEOs can be eliminated by gaining a better understanding of the competitive environment in which hospitals must function. A "business as usual" attitude is no longer appropriate in many markets, and refocusing attention and talents on developing competitive strategies is the first step toward a hospital's long-term stability and success. An evaluation of the internal forces affecting a hospital's strategic decision-making process, combined with an evaluation of external forces affecting the hospital (as discussed in chapter 2), is the basis for the development of a competitive strategy.

This chapter identifies the internal factors that a hospital executive should analyze prior to contracting with health maintenance organizations (HMOs), preferred provider organizations (PPOs), and employers. It discusses the need for organizational and governance structures that allow for competitive flexibility; the hospital's mission and goals as they relate to competitive goals and operating policies; the hospital's image and perceived reputation; development of products and product lines that are responsive to competitive forces; medical staff profiling; short-term and long-term investments in technology; financial issues related to employer, PPO, and HMO contracting; and administrative staff capabilities and skills that are required for competitive contracting.

Hospital Structure and Governance

To operate competitively and to contract effectively with HMOs, PPOs, and employers, a hospital must be part of a comprehensive and flexible organizational and governance structure. Although a particular structure is not advocated here, the structure adopted must be flexible enough to allow the hospital chief executive officer (CEO) or the individual with designated responsibility to evaluate and respond quickly to various contracting opportunities.

A hospital organizational structure that is useful in contracting arrangements is one that is flexible and is designed with separate operating divisions having different functions, product lines, and purposes. These divisions may be organized as separate legal entities if such an organization is required by the hospital's strategic objectives. Such a structure usually consists of a parent corporation with not-for-profit and for-profit subsidiaries developed as necessary. Subsidiaries can also include partnership arrangements with medical practitioners to facilitate contracting for full or specialty services.

The hospital may choose to develop separate legal entities for a number of reasons, including avoidance of restrictions associated with not-for-profit status, increased access to financial resources, and enhancement of flexibility in its decision-making ability. Any organizational structure implemented by a hospital involved in or planning for contracting should also allow various service units to be marketed, priced, and operated relatively independently.

The hospital CEO must recognize the constraints and advantages of these organizational structures. Not clearly delineating who has authority to make key decisions can impair the hospital's ability to operate effectively in a competitive marketplace. Personnel selected to head each corporate entity must be given appropriate decision-making authority so that they can effectively take advantage of any competitive opportunity that may arise.

The hospital CEO should be cognizant not only of the impact of the internal governance structure of the hospital but also of the hospital's position within its broader corporate organizational and governance structure. For example, many hospitals are a part of regional or national organizational frameworks that delegate different levels of authority to the hospital. To be avoided is a situation in which the hospital CEO may have inadvertently conveyed the wrong impression of his or her level of authority and consequently enters into competitive arrangements only to have to alter them at the direction of corporate staff.

Some competitive opportunities can be best addressed at the local level and do not lend themselves to effective centralized corporate control. When faced with these situations, the local CEO must be able to assume greater responsibility in order to respond competitively. The hospital's strategic plan and mission and goals statements should provide the CEO with the direction needed to manage these situations.

Today's CEOs find themselves surrounded by various corporate structures and interrelationships that require increased administrative skills but also offer the corporate support that is needed to compete in today's health care environment. In preparing for contracting, the pros and cons of all potential organizational structures and affiliations must be carefully analyzed.

Mission and Goals

Before a hospital can enter today's competitive marketplace through contracting, the CEO should thoroughly analyze the organization's mission and goals to ensure that any developed competitive strategies are consistent with its mission and goals. For example, many church-sponsored hospitals may have a mission of serving the poor in their communities. Realizing that this mission statement may conflict with the reality of remaining financially solvent, some of these hospitals have had to revise their mission statements to accommodate the demands of a competitive marketplace. In 1983, as part of a competitive strategy, one church-sponsored hospital developed a hospital-based PPO. The strategy involved revising the hospital's mission and goals to reflect the intent to provide competitive options for employers seeking to contain health care costs. When an institution is competitively positioned, the mission and goals must reflect a corporate philosophy that can often balance two potentially opposing forces.

Image

The hospital's image is an important factor in contracting with HMOs, PPOs, and employers. Image is generally built on such aspects as the internal and external appearance of the physical plant; the location and ease of access to the facility; and the community's historical perceptions of the quality of the medical staff, nursing staff, and administration. Image also includes the community's perception of the hospital's charges for the services rendered; that is, a hospital may be regarded by the community as a "high-priced" institution even though the average cost per stay is in line or below the averages for the community. Improving a hospital's negative reputation can be a difficult and time-consuming task that requires communication and marketing sophistication.

Hospital management should consider the institution's image as it is viewed not only by potential and former patients but also by the business community. What is the hospital's reputation among insurance carriers and operating HMOs and PPOs? Is the institution thought to have a utilization or quality assurance problem? Is it perceived to have a poorly trained medical staff? Such an evaluation from the perspective of the group purchaser is of key importance. A marketing consulting firm may be able to provide assistance if hospital management does not believe it has accurate knowledge of the institution's true reputation in the community.

A hospital often enjoys financial gains when it has a community reputation for high-quality services. For example, one urban hospital found that it did not have to discount services to obtain a contract with HMOs and PPOs because it was already perceived as a cost-effective, high-quality institution. Another hospital was not so fortunate. It had previously used questionable treatment programs that came under public scrutiny. Ten years later, this hospital is still struggling to overcome the adverse publicity and its negative effect in contracting situations.

Just as a hospital should realistically examine, and strive to alter as necessary, its image and reputation, so should it examine the reputation of groups with whom it chooses to affiliate via contracts. Not all affiliations are viewed as positive competitive alliances. Affiliations should enhance the market positions of both parties and strengthen their combined efforts. If this strengthening of positions does not occur, the affiliation should be avoided. Several excellent hospitals have damaged their favorably perceived reputations by contracting with insurance carriers, other hospitals, and HMOs with lesser reputations.

A hospital should not enter into any contracting situation without first considering the effect of that alliance on its reputation and image. Although image has historically been important to hospitals, it now becomes increasingly important in a competitive market. To improve its image, a hospital may need to make administrative and medical staff changes, renovate or relocate its physical plant, or add or eliminate some offered medical services.

Product Definition

To compete in today's marketplace, hospitals need to look at their patient care services as separate and distinct product lines rather than as a broad collection of individual services, as has been the practice. For example, the individual services of breast cancer screening, osteoporosis screening, stress management, and weight reduction classes should be regarded as a comprehensive program aimed at women. A marketing strategy should be specifically designed to promote these services as a product line.

Management should determine which services distinguish the hospital from other competing institutions in the community and then decide to whom the services should be marketed. Such a market-identification analysis is important because it helps the hospital to ascertain administrative support needs and to develop a program to promote the product. Then the hospital should examine the various components of the product to decide if any additional staffing and resources are required. Because the hospital's products are an integral part of the strategic plan for contracting with HMOs, PPOs, and employers, the hospital should determine how each product line fits into the short-term and long-term plan for external contracting, associated pricing arrangements, and potential profitability.

Medical Staff

Physician recruitment is an area requiring close analysis by hospital CEOs. Are the hospital's physician recruitment practices consistent with its competitive philosophy? A hospital may have a goal of attracting private-pay patients. Therefore, the hospital's medical staff should have a sufficient mix of specialty and primary care physicians whose offices are located in an area near the residences of the targeted patient population. A hospital with an overabundance of specialty physicians may need to recruit a larger complement of primary care physicians if it wishes to contract with HMOs or PPOs. To accomplish these changes, a hospital may have to reconsider current services, programs, or cost structures as well as assessments of and revisions to current medical staff recruitment criteria.

Hospital management should not overlook the significance of its medical staff in the strategic planning for contracting with PPOs, HMOs, and employers. The attitudes of the medical staff should be compatible with the goals of the organization. One hospital system worked closely with consultants to develop a hospital-based PPO program. During a meeting with a group of key physicians four months into the process, hospital administration learned that as a result of rumors that had been circulating among the medical staff for months, the majority of physicians felt threatened and were adamantly opposed to participating in this joint venture with the hospital. Avoiding this type of situation is essential.

Before embarking on a competitive strategy that includes physician involvement, hospital administration should evaluate its medical staff in terms of:

- *Physician profiling and practice patterns.* Physicians' patients are reviewed by diagnosis-related group (DRG), and the actual length of stay (LOS) of those patients is compared with Medicare and hospital norms. The hospital's average charges per DRG are compared with the Medicare reimbursed amount per DRG, and the variance is shown. The following information by physician should be collected:
  - Description of DRG treated
  - DRG number
  - Number of patients treated under each DRG by specific physician
  - Medicare's and hospital's average LOS for each DRG treated
  - Average LOS by specific physician for each DRG treated
  - Variances between Medicare's and the hospital's averages and the average LOS by specific physician for each DRG treated
  - Actual amount paid by Medicare or the average of the actual charges for all physicians treating this DRG
  - Average of actual charges by specific physician for each DRG treated
  - Variance between the actual amount paid by Medicare or the average of the actual charges for all physicians treating this DRG and the average by specific physician of actual charges for each DRG treated by that physician
- *Individual physician's share of hospital admissions and service utilization.* The potential loss of admissions to the hospital if the physician admits elsewhere should be determined.
- *Physician involvement with HMOs, individual practice associations (IPAs), or PPOs.* A physician involved with one of these groups may be more accustomed to certain utilization management practices. Also, physicians may have an exclusive contract with an organization.

- *Average age of the medical staff.* Younger physicians may be more receptive to changes in their medical practice than are those who have established practices.
- *Medical staff mix.* The hospital should have a sufficient complement of primary care physicians as well as specialty physicians.
- *The reputation of the medical staff.* The institution should have a significant number of physicians who are well-known and well-respected in the community.
- *Recruitment.* The hospital should have on its medical staff physicians who can serve as good recruiters for other desired physicians.

Physicians must play a key role in issues such as utilization management and peer review. However, hospital management should be aware of issues that cannot directly involve physicians. For example, physicians should not be involved in determining physician fee schedules in contracting arrangements because of potential conflicts with price fixing and antitrust regulations. One hospital that was developing a joint-venture PPO contracting entity with its medical staff initially included physicians in fee discussions. When a legal consultant advised the hospital management that physicians could be subject to charges of price fixing, the physicians were asked to resign from committees that were considering pricing data. This situation indicates that, in this case at least, hospital administration must be well informed regarding legal issues.

Hospital management should be sensitive to the impact that strategic competitive planning can have on physicians who choose not to participate. The hospital should avoid alienating nonparticipating physicians and allowing a negative political situation to arise among physicians on staff. Clear communication and open and honest collaboration early in the process foster a strong working relationship with the institution's medical staff.

Technology

Hospitals need to assess the likely effects of future demand for specific hospital services that are associated with advances in technology. The introduction of complex diagnostic technology may either increase inpatient services or may actually decrease patient days by shifting delivery from the inpatient to the outpatient setting. Anesthetic and surgical advances may increase the use of outpatient surgery, and pharmacologic and medical treatments may replace surgery and other invasive forms of therapy. Ongoing assessments need to be made of the potential shift in hospital volume that may be associated with these and other technological changes.

Insurance coverage usually lags behind the development of new medical procedures made possible by technological breakthroughs. Often payers define new procedures as experimental or as lacking therapeutic value. Payers and their customers may also be cautious about the medical and financial efficiency of the new services. Hospital management should be aware of these implications when considering new technology. Another concern expressed by payers is that new technology does not necessarily lower the cost of health care.

A hospital must maintain an acceptable level of new technology if it is to remain attractive to its medical staff as well as to organizations with which it may contract in the future. The purchase of new technology should be an integral part of the institution's goals. A flexible organizational structure, as mentioned earlier, can help hospital management avoid political and governmental roadblocks to the acquisition of appropriate new technology.

Finances

Hospitals striving for true competitive strength assess the marketability of their services and products as viewed by the consumer. As a result, the issue of price-competitive products as related to the cost of the product is now a major focus in a hospital's financial analysis. Hospitals must take a look at the financial issues that may influence their decision about contracting: pricing and payer mix, employer analysis of costs, financial profiling, uncompensated care, and financial monitoring systems.

Pricing and Payer Mix

Typically, a complex interrelationship exists between what it costs a hospital to provide services and what the hospital charges various categories of patients for services. The ability to charge for services relates to a variety of existing financial arrangements with government

(Medicare, Medicaid, and others); negotiated rates with various organizations; and hospital-determined charges, which are primarily for private payers, including third-party commercial insurance carriers. An evaluation of these financial arrangements and related charges is helpful in determining whether or not charges are competitive.

Figure 1-1 shows how a hospital's pricing structure relates to various categories of payers. Historically, government reimbursement for Medicare and Medicaid recipients has been insufficient to cover expenses incurred by the hospital for these individuals. Consequently, unrecovered hospital costs were shifted to the private-pay sector, as indicated in figure 1-1. In addition, hospitals are not reimbursed for their bad debt or charity cases, and so these costs are also shifted to private payers. Therefore, the private-payer charges cover costs, including shifted unrecovered costs and a predetermined profit margin. In figure 1-1, the subject hospital's payer mix consists of 55 percent private payers (or full-pay charges), 5 percent bad debt and charity, 10 percent Medicaid, and 30 percent Medicare.

Further complicating a hospital's problem of maintaining an adequate margin between revenues and expenses is the shrinking number of patients who pay full charges. Many of these patients are joining HMOs and PPOs, which usually reimburse the hospital at less than full charges but generally more than cost. Negotiated reimbursement from HMOs, PPOs, and direct employer contracts results in fewer private-sector payers to whom shifted costs can be distributed (figure 1-2). Also eroding the profitability of a hospital's patient base is the trend toward performing more procedures on an outpatient basis and charging less for them. All of these competitive programs are shown as negotiated patients in figure 1-2. Competitive pricing for HMOs, PPOs, and direct employer contracts becomes more difficult as the number of private-sector payers continues to shrink, resulting in a smaller base over which to shift unrecovered costs. Figure 1-2 shows a payer base shift to 40 percent full-pay charges and 15 percent negotiated charges.

Management should analyze the hospital's pricing strategy to determine if prices are competitive for its service area. In developing pricing strategies and proposals, hospitals should consider the actual costs of providing services, expected utilization levels and severity of illness for both current and future patients, value and collectibility of patient deductibles and coinsurance, and the payment methods

Figure 1-1. Hospital Financial Constraints: Cost Reimbursement and Full-Pay Charges

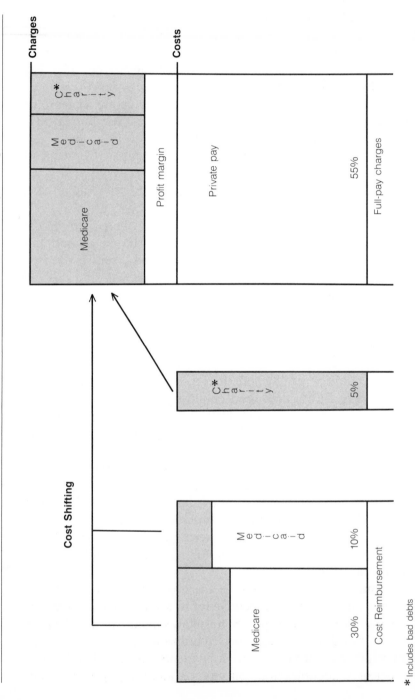

* Includes bad debts

Figure 1-2. Hospital Financial Constraints: Negotiated, Cost Reimbursement, and Full-Pay Charges

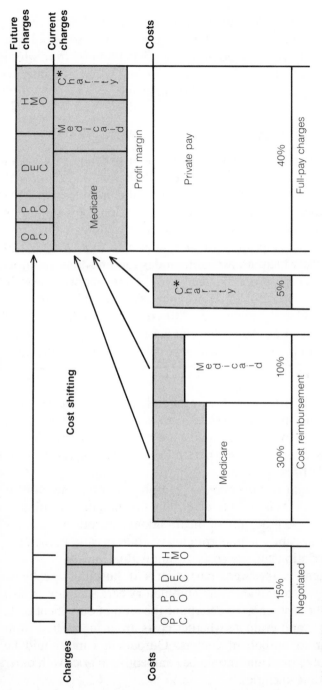

Key to abbreviations:
OPC—outpatient care
PPO—preferred provider organizations
DEC—direct employer contracts
HMO—health maintenance organizations

*Includes bad debts

used by group purchasers. The effect on the current patient load of not contracting with PPOs, HMOs, or employers also should be assessed. The final results should provide a pricing strategy from which a hospital can evaluate proposed programs and associated rates to determine if they can be successfully managed.

Employer Analysis of Costs

Hospitals should be aware that employers seeking to contract for health care services use available claims data on admissions and charges of community hospitals that serve the majority of employees under the employers' medical benefits plans. This information helps employers to determine utilization trends and make charge comparisons.

Other tools that employers use in evaluating hospitals are Medicare cost reports, which are available under the Freedom of Information Act. When properly analyzed, these reports provide information that is useful in determining contractual approaches between payer and individual hospital. By reviewing each report and abstracting key data elements, the purchaser can formulate strategies for negotiations with individual providers. The key data provided are as follows:

- *Financial profitability.* A careful review of the balance sheet and income and expense statements shows the profitability of the hospital. A review of a hospital's accounts receivable and other asset items can help determine the aggressiveness of the hospital's fiscal policies.
- *Ancillary and routine charges.* Simply reviewing the ratio of costs to charges in total to determine the margin of profitability is insufficient because of the traditional overpricing of ancillary services and the underpricing of routine care. Rather, the charge relationship to costs by individual ancillary service department is reviewed, particularly if hospitals are being encouraged to provide more ambulatory care. Employers also look at the cost report to determine the ratio of outpatient costs to charges and evaluate whether costs are being shifted from inpatient to outpatient centers. Outpatient care should be reasonably priced and should be competitive in price with other freestanding facilities.

- *Patient mix.* The financial flexibility of a hospital, which is limited by the financial mix of its patients, can affect negotiating strength. The higher the private-pay mix, the more profitable a facility should be. Many hospitals consider a 55 percent private-pay mix ideal because government programs have traditionally reimbursed less than full costs.

Another source of information readily accessible to employers is charge data from both health care coalitions and government-sponsored groups such as the Illinois Health Care Cost Containment Council. These groups publish and disseminate average hospital per diem and other charge data. However, the information is not as detailed or reliable as that available from internal sources or Medicare cost reports.

Information on hospital charge data is also available from business coalitions and user groups. The Midwest Business Group on Health and other coalitions encourage employers to share the information they have on hospitals, including data on hospital charges derived from submitted claims. The Washington Business Group on Health has a well-established reputation for assisting employers in obtaining hospital-specific information.

As an employer, the hospital can also look at its own employee health care claims data to determine its own price competitiveness. Through this analysis of its employee claims data, a hospital can determine what competitors are charging its employees for various services and then compare the competitors' charges with its own. Outside help may be needed in case mix adjustment and comparison to normative data.

Financial Profiling

The hospital should develop a comprehensive internal financial profile. To develop this profile, the hospital must collect and analyze information on the following:

- Patient charge data.
- Profitability by DRG.
- Profitability by patient mix.
- Profitability by physician.

- Cost per service.
- Analysis of major payers (further defined by group purchaser, for example, employer name, Taft-Hartley Trust Fund, or other). This analysis should include which physicians treat these employers' employees and the major diagnosis categories of the persons treated.

After the hospital develops its profile, it should examine it carefully to see if the hospital has the service capability to make strategic program changes in response to any long-term trends that are related to specific purchasers who are of key importance to the institution. Both government and private third-party payers are particularly interested in contracting with hospitals that can provide health care services in a cost-effective manner.

The following financial questions or issues should be addressed before any contractual relationship with a major purchaser is finalized. Analysis should be based on the outcome of financial profiling and strategy development.

- What are the expected revenue increases from new patients attracted to the hospital because of the contract?
- What is the anticipated shift of current full-pay patients to contract patients?
- If the hospital does not contract, what is the anticipated loss of revenue from decreased utilization by existing patients who may enroll in the new contracted program?
- What is the revenue-decrease level associated with existing full-charge patients who may enroll in new contracted programs and receive care under negotiated-rate arrangements?
- What are the maximum and minimum revenue and expenses related to risk-sharing contracts?
- What additional operating-cost increases will result from the new contractual arrangements and the associated administrative tasks involved?

Uncompensated Care

Uncompensated care costs are an important factor that hospitals must carefully consider when preparing for contracting. This subject, which requires extensive discussion with third-party payers, should be raised early in the negotiation process. The uncompensated care issue is critical because various federal and state programs often do not reimburse for total costs and therefore are contributors to the uncompensated care problem.

Careful, detailed explanations are required to ensure a thorough understanding of uncompensated care on the part of the purchaser. However, such discussion cannot occur unless hospitals document levels of uncompensated costs prior to contracting and develop a strategy for negotiations based on this knowledge.

A formula should be developed to distribute an appropriate share of the uncompensated costs to purchasers. This formula can be a ratio using patient days, revenue dollars, admissions, or any other appropriate index. Many purchasers realize their commitment to these costs and are attempting to develop acceptable ways of sharing them.

Data Monitoring Systems

Once a contract is in force, the hospital needs financial systems that are capable of monitoring patients involved in negotiated arrangements on a daily basis and of aggregating utilization data. Hospital management needs to review these data to ensure that the purchaser complies with negotiated contracts and the negotiated rates remain profitable. At minimum, hospitals need a system that can gather the information shown in figure 1-3 for all patients covered by special contracted rates.

Census report formats, such as that shown in figure 1-4 should include such variables as the patient's name, room number, type of accommodation, daily rate, account number, sex, contracting code (that is, HMO affiliation), attending physician, date of admission, and accumulated balance. For example, figure 1-4 indicates that Marie Smith is affiliated with Good Health HMO (code 3) and her accumulated hospital charges through July 2, 1987, are $3,081. This record can be compared with the HMO contract to show any financial risk being assumed by the hospital. Patients Baler and Allen were covered by the employer PPO (code 1) and are being reimbursed on a per diem basis.

Close daily monitoring of patients receiving services through contract arrangements gives the hospital the opportunity to exchange utilization data with purchasers. The purchaser report shown in figure 1-5 compares the contract fee to the actual fee for each inpatient by

Figure 1-3.   Minimum Data Elements

Patient information
Birth date
Sex
Relationship to insured
ZIP code
Patient identification number
Claim number

Insured information
Social Security number or employee number
Insurance number
Employee status (active, retired, and so forth)
Sex
Birth date
Insurance group or indicator of type of benefit plan

Hospital information
Hospital name
Federal tax number
Hospital ZIP code

Physician
Name of physician

Federal tax number of admitting physician
Federal tax number of attending physician
Federal tax number of surgeon

Employer
Location
Identification

Payer
Identification

Admission
Date
Type (emergency, urgent, elective, newborn)
Source (emergency department, physician, acute hospital, skilled nursing facility, and so forth)
Hour

Discharge
Date
Disposition (home, skilled nursing facility, died, and so forth)

Clinical
Coding system—diagnosis (for example, ICD-9-CM)

Principal diagnosis
Secondary diagnosis
Coding system—procedure (for example, ICD-9-CM, CPT-4)
Principal procedure
Date of principal procedure
Secondary procedures
Date of secondary procedures

Claim administration
Type of bill (final, interim)
Service
Place of service
Condition codes

Charge
Dates indicating period covered by statement
Total amount of charge
Deductible
Coinsurance
Amount paid
Prior payment
Coordination of benefits
Service code and charge

Figure 1-4. Example of a Census Report

ABC Hospital
Selected Census Report

Page 1
07/31/87

Room No.	Type of Accommodation	Daily Rate	Patient Name	Account Number	Sex	Contract Code	Attending Physician	Admission Date	Accumulated Balance
1201	Prvt	$183	Smith, Marie	44872643	F	3	Young, T.	06/29/87	$ 3,081
635	Semi	$165	Baler, Wilbur	83134261	M	1	Smith, W.	07/01/87	$ 386
905	ICU	$375	Allen, Don	55468004	M	1	Penn, D.	06/15/87	$27,286

Copyright 1987, William M. Mercer-Meidinger-Hansen. Reproduction in whole or in part is permissible with credit to William M. Mercer-Meidinger-Hansen.

Figure 1-5. Example of a Patient Analysis by Purchaser Group

ABC Hospital
Employer Association, Inc.
Patient Analysis

Page 1
07/31/87

Patient Number	Admission Date	DRG	Surgical Procedure	Standard LOS	Actual LOS	Contract Fee	Actual Fee
44872643	06/29/87	Bronchitis	—	4.1	4.0	$ 2,545	$ 3,081
55468004	06/15/87	Pulmonary embolism	—	12.1	8.0	$10,565	$ 6,832
83134261	07/01/87	Rhinoplasty	Septoplasty	3.1	2.0	$ 1,208	$ 1,042
	Totals			6.4	4.7	$14,318	$10,955

Copyright 1987, William M. Mercer-Meidinger-Hansen. Reproduction in whole or in part is permissible with credit to William M. Mercer-Meidinger-Hansen.

DRG or surgical procedure. This report allows a purchaser to compare the value of the negotiated contract with actual performance to determine the effectiveness of the contract. This kind of working arrangement requires effective data monitoring and a willingness on the part of the provider to work with purchasers.

If hospitals contract to provide reports to purchasers, they should in turn receive reports from purchasers profiling the hospital's performance and market share. The example of this type of report, shown in figure 1-6, is an indication of the hospital's share of the purchaser's market, its charges, and the severity of illness of patients compared with those treated by competing providers. This report also compares one hospital with a peer hospital and shows how the hospital fared in a given quarter, year to date, and the previous year. Comparative peer-hospital data are evaluated by such variables as average charge per stay and per day, average LOS, and the severity of patient illness as determined by the hospital's DRG cost weights. These data are the key to monitoring hospital performance in contracted arrangements.

Figure 1-6. Example of a Provider Profile by Purchaser Group

	Employer Association, Inc. ABC Hospital Provider Profile		Page 1 07/31/87
Services summary	**Current Quarter**	**Year to Date**	**Last Year**
Admissions	276	1,543	722
Total patient days	1,300	6,172	3,088
Market share	25%	30%	15%
Patient demographics	25	20	10
	ABC Hospital		**Peer Hospital**
Average charge per stay	$2,880		$4,699
Average charge per day	$ 576		$ 723
Average LOS	5.0		6.5
Patient severity	1.023		.9846

Administrative Staff

When planning for HMO, PPO, and employer contracting, hospitals need to consider their administrative expertise. An assessment and understanding of needed talent should be undertaken by hospital management. Staff members skilled in the following areas are essential:

- *Finance.* The financial staff should be experienced in pricing hospital services competitively and should be familiar with the hospital's data management capability. They should have the expertise to accurately assess the risks involved in contracting with employers, HMOs, and PPOs. This process may require actuarial assistance before risk contracts are finalized if the potential risk to be assumed is to be fully evaluated.
- *Marketing.* The marketing staff should be acquainted with key business decision makers in the community. Knowledge of the strengths of the competition and the competition's financial base is important. Marketing staff should know how to develop a marketing strategy that promotes individual hospital services within the community (product-line marketing).
- *Legal.* Legal staff should be experienced in the development of different types of partnership and joint-venture arrangements and in contract development and evaluation. They should also be familiar with relevant state and federal laws and regulations.
- *Utilization management.* The individuals managing utilization and quality assurance programs should be well regarded by the medical staff. The utilization management staff should be able to do case analysis on both Medicare and private-pay patients or any patients covered by contracts with shared risks.
- *Contract negotiation.* A member of the hospital's administrative staff should be able to negotiate contracts with HMOs, PPOs, and employers in consultation with legal staff. This individual should be skilled in developing negotiating strategies and should have a thorough knowledge of the medical services delivery capability of the hospital.
- *Health benefits design.* Hospital management may find it helpful to include on the team an individual who is familiar with the design of health benefits plans. Understanding employer

needs and benefits can prove helpful to a hospital in determining which medical services to offer to employers.

Many current hospital staff members may be able to perform these functions. However, additional staff with new skills or experience may be required, depending on the local marketplace and the level of competition.

Conclusion

Essential for the creation of a competitive nucleus is a flexible yet comprehensive corporate structure that allows freedom to respond to competitive situations. Clear corporate goals and positive marketing images give hospitals a direction in developing services that are desired by the local community. Hospitals must begin to realize that through proper physician recruitment and planning, they can influence their future patient mix and financial success.

Financial flexibility is important to the success of any marketing endeavor. A close working relationship between the medical staff and the administrative staff is an absolute requirement for delivering a total package of competitive services.

Chapter 2

Evaluating External Forces

Introduction

Preparing for contracting relationships requires a thorough evaluation of external forces affecting hospitals in addition to the evaluation of internal forces discussed in chapter 1. Although hospitals have traditionally evaluated such aspects periodically, the needs of an increasingly competitive environment create new urgency and require more concentrated and ongoing evaluations of the forces affecting the hospital. Newly evolving competitive pricing approaches and consumer choice are altering previous planning and evaluation processes. Chapter 2 focuses on evaluating general marketplace characteristics, risk sharing, and regulatory and legal issues.

Marketplace Characteristics

An assessment of the marketplace includes gathering and evaluating data on consumers, payers, and other providers within the community. This market research leads ultimately to defining the hospital's potential market share and competition and initiates the process of defining the hospital's strategy for developing relationships with purchasers.

Community Demographics

Determining the prevalence of demographic characteristics that support the implementation of contracting approaches requires the analysis of a variety of data. Because hospitals have traditionally evaluated these factors on a limited basis (for example, patient origin by ZIP code), they may need only to expand their efforts and alter the framework of the data.

An examination of community census data and the relationship of these data to the hospital's patient mix can be useful in developing contracting strategy. Census data can be displayed according to ZIP code, age, sex, economic status, household size, and other readily available statistics. This information, along with assumptions on payer source, service utilization patterns, and future trends, can help the hospital determine service requirements and appropriate marketing approaches. For example, if the data show that the hospital's target population consists of a high proportion of women of childbearing years or the elderly, it can expect to have higher than average rates of admissions for childbirth and female reproductive disorders or for chronic diseases. Therefore, the hospital should develop its product mix to incorporate services for women or the elderly.

Several community demographic characteristics are pertinent indicators for the success of preferred provider organizations (PPOs), health maintenance organizations (HMOs), or other managed care plans. An assessment of the characteristics of members of PPOs and HMOs in the hospital's market area in combination with the demographic characteristics of the overall market helps focus the hospital's strategy. A hospital that finds its market to consist of young, mobile, employed persons with larger households may consider participating in an HMO because persons interested in using an HMO may have specific characteristics, as shown in figure 2-1.

After assessing community demographics, one hospital found that the median age of its target population was rapidly decreasing because of an influx of new industry. Further, this population was interested in convenience services because of the large number of working mothers. This analysis combined with others led the hospital to conclude that it should seek contracting relationships with HMOs and PPOs and that it should develop specific convenience services, such as urgent care services and care offered after regular business hours. Another hospital determined that the median age of the population in its market area was increasing, primarily because younger residents were not remaining in the area. This hospital decided to contract in the future with competitive medical plans (CMPs) to attract Medicare recipients and is currently developing services geared to an older population.

A further evaluation of community demographics, combined with actuarial analysis, enables a hospital to preliminarily project hospital admissions and utilization trends for the population. A comparison of these data with the hospital's actual experience and with the experiences of other area hospitals provides a picture of correct market share and a projection of future market share.

Payer Sources and Requirements

Hospitals involved in the development of competitive strategies should identify their predominant purchaser sources, or employers, in the hospital's current and potential market area. Once the hospital knows who the key employers are, it can then evaluate them in terms of the following:

- Amount of charges incurred at the hospital over a 12-month period

Figure 2-1. Characteristics of HMO Members

Members under 65	
Characteristics	**Reasons for Joining**
No satisfactory relationship with primary physician	Broad scope of benefits
Newer to area	Location of services
Use health services significantly less or more	Expect lower expenses
Younger	Ensured access
Larger families	Administrative ease
Younger children	
Lower income (but employed)	

Members over 65	
Characteristics	**Reasons for Joining**
No satisfactory relationship with primary physician	Broad scope of benefits
Use health services significantly less or more	Location of services
Younger in age group	Expect lower expenses
Fixed income	Ensured access
	Administrative ease

- Current medical-plan funding mechanisms (self-insured, fully insured, minimum premium, and so forth)
- Cost containment strategies already applied or planned
- Interest in PPO, HMO, or direct hospital affiliations

Such information is useful to the hospital as it develops a strategy for negotiating with current and prospective purchasers.

Hospitals currently contracting with HMOs and PPOs should examine the percentage of total admissions that these organizations represent. The decision to continue contracting with current PPOs and HMOs is directly associated with the impact of that purchaser on total admissions and with the hospital's goals and competitive contracting strategy. For example, one hospital determined that a single HMO was responsible for 90 percent of its admissions. The hospital decided to contract with other HMOs in the community to spread its sources of admissions. Depending on one HMO for admissions can be an unwise contracting strategy because of potential political and financial pressures that the HMO can exert on the hospital.

The hospital also should determine profitability by payer source. As mentioned in chapter 1, one source of profitability information by payer is an analysis of the hospital's own data. The hospital should further segregate payer information to determine the top 10 to 20 employers whose employees use hospital services and analyze each of these employers on a cost-to-charge basis to see if these arrangements are cost-effective and should be capitalized on or if additional purchaser sources should be sought. For example, if the hospital is profitably providing services to the elderly population through a contract with a local HMO, it should expand those lines of services that appeal to this patient population. When one hospital analyzed its private-pay sources, it discovered that the employees, beneficiaries, and retirees of one manufacturer represented about 53 percent of all admissions to the hospital. This profitable purchasing organization was targeted for further examination.

In performing market research, the hospital should also survey employers directly to gather detailed information from those employers currently utilizing the facility as well as employers who are located close to the hospital but whose employees do not use the facility. The survey should include a cross section of retail, wholesale, service, government, manufacturing, and other industry types. Further, all sizes of employers, from 25 employees up, should be included.

Employers should be asked questions about the following:

- Their perception of health care costs and quality of care provided
- Medical plan funding, which includes information about the employer's funding arrangement, relationship with insurance brokerage firms, and the general structure and design of their benefits plan
- Additional services desired from providers
- Historical cost of providing health care benefits to employees
- Current cost containment activities
- Perceptions of how well HMOs and PPOs work to contain costs and ensure high-quality care
- Perception of the hospital relative to its competition

Once collected and analyzed, the survey data should be an integral part of a competitive strategic plan. The survey data provide the hospital with valuable information for establishing priorities with regard to contracting methods and for targeting influential employers, who may be interested in negotiating arrangements with hospitals that are major providers of health care services for their employees. Using the information provided by the survey, hospitals should be able to determine which employers have experienced substantial increases in their health care premiums, which have cost-shifted copayments or deductibles to their employees, and which have incorporated cost containment strategies such as outpatient surgery and second-surgical-opinion programs into their benefits plans.

Competitive Position

To be able to compete effectively, the hospital must thoroughly understand its competitors. Gathering information through an evaluation of Medicare cost reports or other information sources helps the hospital to better evaluate its competition. Following is a list of data that may be useful in such an evaluation:

- Average occupancy rate
- The hospital's Medicare intensity index
- Cost-to-charge ratios, which indicate the percentage markup
- Contractual allowances (bad debts, charity care, negotiated discounts) and accounts receivable as a percentage of patient revenues
- Total discharges and average charge per discharge
- Payer mix (private-pay patient base, Medicare, Medicaid, and uncompensated care as a percentage of patient days)
- Ratio of costs to charges by ancillary department
- Average inpatient costs and charges
- Hospital balance sheet

This information can also be used by employers to help them evaluate hospitals with whom they want to contract.

As part of the competitive planning and market analysis, hospital management should determine what services competitive organizations offer and what their estimated share of the market is by service. The hospital should decide if it can provide all the services that HMOs, PPOs, and employers may require or if it needs to contract with a competitor for selected services. The short-term and long-term liability of this decision should be considered.

The types of patient services a hospital provides are a direct result of the composition of its medical staff. Careful recruitment of physicians should result in the type of medical staff that meets the hospital's goals, as discussed in chapter 1.

Risk-Sharing Arrangements

Risk-sharing arrangements spread financial risk among the employer, employee, and provider. The purpose of negotiating risk arrangements is to place all parties at some level of financial risk for the cost of services delivered. Employers are placed at risk through self-funding and various types of premium participation. Employers may also be placed at risk if they choose to contract directly with providers or offer incentives for employees to use specific providers. Employees are placed at risk through benefits plan incentives and freedom of choice. Risk sharing is viewed by many purchasers as an attractive cost-management strategy. It can also work to a hospital's advantage if it is appropriately understood, calculated, and negotiated by the hospital.

The concept of risk sharing between providers and purchasers is likely to attract wide purchaser support because it signals accountability for the cost of health care. Major participants in contracting for health care need to carefully consider all the basic assumptions of any financial arrangements and thoroughly understand what they are contracting for. Different points of view need to be clarified before and during the negotiation process so that purchasers and providers can develop mutual trust and long-term relationships.

Any financial risks shared with employers, PPOs, or HMOs should be in proportion to the financial incentives given by the purchaser in directing employees and subscribers to the hospital. The objective is to establish mutual trust based on good-faith actions from all parties in the contracting process. General guidelines for incentives versus level of risk assumed should be developed during the hospital's strategic planning process.

To determine the amount of risk an employer will assume, the hospital must understand how the size of the employee group affects the level of risk that an employer can handle. For example, businesses of 15 to 300 employees are often fully insured, and so the employer assumes no risk. The medium to large employers (200 to 700 employees) often assume slightly more risk by choosing minimum-premium arrangements. In these arrangements, the employer pays the insurance company a reduced premium every month, and the employer and insurance company balance the remainder of the claims billing due at the end of the year and credit any overpayments. Self-insured options, which are usually reserved for larger employers, give the employer the greatest amount of cash flow but also entail a higher degree of risk. In these self-insured arrangements, the claims administrator simply pays claims and issues reports describing the employer's claims experience. Self-insured employers decrease risk through the purchase of stop-loss insurance on a per occurrence or aggregate basis.

An employer's ability to benefit from PPO or direct contracting relationships is dependent on these insurance arrangements. The greater the employers' risk, the more they can benefit from contracting. Hospitals should consider this fact when evaluating major purchasers.

Hospital management should understand the ramifications of risk sharing and different payment methodologies and of risk sharing through pooling arrangements. Figure 2-2 describes payment methods and the hospital risk associated with their effect on admissions, LOS, use of ancillary services, and case mix. For example, if a hospital chooses a single per diem payment method, a change in its admissions rate is not a factor in determining risk, but a change in case mix becomes critical because the payment is on a per diem basis. In a combination of per case and per diem payment, the physician's use of ancillary services places the hospital at full risk because payment is related to fixed per case or per diem amounts. The change in case mix places the hospital at limited financial risk if per diem payments relate to all case types.

Figure 2-3 indicates several payment options for hospitals and physicians. This figure details data requirements for setting initial

Figure 2-2. Hospital Provider Payment Options and Related Risk

Payment Option	Change in Admissions	Change in LOS	Usage of Ancillary Services	Change in Case Mix
Standard charges	No risk to HSA	No risk	No risk	No risk
Discounted charges	No risk	No risk	No risk	No risk
Per diem rates	No risk	Limited risk	Full risk	Full risk
Combination of per case and per diem rates	Limited risk	Limited risk	Full risk	Limited risk
Single case rate for all cases	No risk	Full risk	Full risk	Full risk
Combination of per case and per diem rates plus performance bonus	Limited risk	Full risk	Full risk	Full risk
Capitation	Full risk	Full risk	Full risk	Full risk

Figure 2-3. Provider Payment Options for Provider Contracts

Range of Risk	Hospital or Other Institutional Service Payment Methods	Pricing and Monitoring Data Needed		Physician Payment Methods	Pricing and Monitoring Data Needed	
		Pricing*	Monitoring†		Pricing*	Monitoring†
No economic risk	Standard charges	1	1,2	Standard charges	1,7	1,2,3
	Discounted charges	1,2	1,2,3	Discounted charges	1,7	1,2,3
	Per diem rates	2,3,4	1,2,4	Reasonable and customary limits by procedure	1,7	1,2,3
	Combination of per case and charges	1,2,3,4,5	1,2,4,5,6	Fixed-fee schedule (relative-value scale or by procedure)	1,7,8	1,2,3
	Combination of per case and per diem	1,2,3,4,5	1,2,4,5,6	Fixed-fee schedule with performance bonus‡ or reasonable and customary limits with performance bonus‡	1,6,7,8	1,2,3,7
	Per case rates for all cases	2,4,5	2,5,6			
	Combination of per case charges with performance bonus	1,2,3,4,5,6	1,2,4,5,6,7			
	Combination of per case and per diem with performance bonus	1,2,3,4,5,6	1,2,4,5,6,7			
Full economic risk	Capitation	2,4,5,6	2,7	Capitation	6	7

*Key to pricing data needed:

1. Current fee or charge schedules by procedure or service

2. Financial information on cost shifting or markups

3. Average charges per day for the hospital

4. LOS data by diagnosis for the hospital

5. DRG-based data on current charges and normative charges per case broken out by LOS, routine, or ancillary charge components

6. Actuarial forecast of expected plan costs and utilization rates

7. Frequency tables of prevailing fees by procedure

8. Development of relative value scale

‡Bonus pool created through:
 (a) Payment set aside by providers
 (b) Employer or insurer contribution
 (c) Combination of (a) and (b)

†Key to monitoring data needed:

1. Periodic claims audit of fees charged

2. Utilization evaluation data

3. Periodic audit to evaluate service frequency by diagnosis or principal procedure

4. Data on LOS by diagnosis group

5. Periodic audits of DRG assignment

6. Periodic audits of DRG price assignment

7. Evaluation of utilization patterns against actuarial forecast

prices and for ongoing monitoring purposes. Methodologies are listed in ascending order from least provider risk (standard charges, discounted charges, per diem rates) to greatest provider risk (capitation).

Figure 2-4 describes several examples of risk-sharing arrangements. Scenario 1 of example A shows that the actuarial estimate of an employer's health care costs for a contract year is $1.2 million, assuming the use of contracted providers. The employer's actual cost for

Figure 2-4. Examples of Risk-Sharing Arrangements

Example A. Health Care Services with 10 Percent Corridor

Scenario 1: Actual cost of health care services
for negotiated term services was $2 million.

Actuarial Estimate of Employer Cost	Prospectively Negotiated 10% Shared-Risk Corridor	Remainder of Actual Cost
$1.2 million (employer pays total)	10% of $1.2 million, or $120,000 (provider responsibility)	$680,000 (employer responsibility)

Actual cost to employer is $1,880,000; provider responsible for $120,000.

Scenario 2: Actual cost of heatlh care services
for negotiated term services was $1 million.

Actuarial Estimate of Employer Cost	Shared-Risk Corridor	Employer Savings (Dollars less than Actuarial Estimate)
$1.2 million	10% of $1.2 million, or $120,000 (provider gain)	$80,000

Employer actual cost is $1.2 million; provider gain is $120,000.

Example B. Mental Health Services, Capped-Payment Arrangement

- Actuarial estimate is $235,000 for 42 admissions at 10 days per admission ($400 per day) and 280 office visits at $80 each.

- Provider agrees to provide above services for capped rate of $235,000. Any excess cost is provider's risk.

- Provider at risk to keep inpatient stays at 10 days per admission ($400 per day) and $80 per office visit.

- Employer at risk to keep utilization at or less than 42 admissions and 280 office visits.

health care is $2 million. A 10 percent risk-sharing arrangement was negotiated with the providers. The provider is responsible for 10 percent of the $1.2 million, or $120,000. The employer's health care costs are $2 million minus the $120,000 for a total of $1,880,000. The employer saved $120,000 because of the shared-risk arrangement with the provider. The provider had a $120,000 expense because of the 10 percent sharing of risk.

Scenario 2 of example A, figure 2-4, shows an actuarial estimate for services of $1.2 million. The cost of the services at the end of the term is $1 million. Providers agreed to share in 10 percent of the actuarial estimate ($1.2 million). The employer's cost is $1 million plus $120,000 paid to providers, for a total of $1.12 million. The providers gained $120,000 because of the shared-risk corridor. The employer saved $80,000 ($1.2 million estimate minus $1 million actual cost minus $120,000 shared-risk bonus to providers).

In example B of figure 2-4, mental health service costs are actuarially estimated at $235,000 for 42 admissions at 10 days per admission and 280 office visits. The provider and employer contract for services for $235,000. Providers are at risk to keep utilization at or less than 10 days per admission. Employers are at risk to keep utilization at or less than 42 admissions and 280 office visits. When contracting for total cost per negotiated year, both providers and purchasers are at significant risk.

Risks can also be shared through risk pools that are developed to share risk between providers and purchasers. Contractual arrangements between providers and HMOs, PPOs, or employers may establish risk pools by withholding a percentage of hospital or physician fees paid by the third party. This withhold pool is distributed at the end of a contracted period based on the cost-effectiveness of the providers in general or of individual providers. Risk pools may also be shared with contracting employers when such arrangements are prospectively negotiated.

Regulatory and Legal Issues

Hospitals should be aware of existing and pending or upcoming laws and regulations that may affect their plans either to contract with HMOs, PPOs, or employers. Laws regulating PPOs are changing rapidly. According to *Regulation of Preferred Provider Organizations: A Legal Guide for Hospital Executives,* published by the American Hospital Association in September 1986, 20 states had in effect statutes that specifically address PPOs. The publication states that, for the most part, these statutes are not designed to restrict or regulate the development of PPOs. Rather, these laws aim to eliminate the perceived impediments to the participation in PPOs of third-party payers. These statutes also modify, where necessary, subscriber freedom-of-choice guarantees and prohibitions of unfair discrimination against beneficiaries.

About 95 percent of the states have laws regulating the formation and operation of HMOs. If a PPO has the characteristics of an HMO as described in the state statute, it may be treated as such. In California, for example, the statute takes the position that if a PPO contracts with payers to provide health care services and then contracts with providers to furnish those services, the PPO is subject to regulation as an HMO. In direct employer contracting, state statutes should be analyzed to determine applicability. Generally, regulatory issues are minimal in direct contracting arrangements.

Hospitals may negotiate for prepaid Medicare business by contracting with local federally qualified HMOs or competitive medical plans (CMPs) that have obtained contracts from the Health Care Financing Administration (HCFA) to serve Medicare patients. A survey of HMOs or CMPs in the hospital's community can determine which HMOs and CMPs have received such approval.

The hospital should be aware of legal issues that affect both the facility and physician providers. Physician contracts often have hold-harmless clauses, which usually state that the physician is solely responsible for malpractice when treating a patient covered by the contract and hold the purchaser harmless. As a result, many malpractice insurers refuse to write insurance for these physicians. Chapter 3 discusses legal issues relating to managed care plans.

Conclusion

This chapter examines external forces that hospital management must evaluate in developing competitive strategies. These forces include community demographics, payer sources and requirements, competitive position, and regulatory requirements.

Combining internal and external evaluation processes can culminate in the development of detailed contracting plans based on the hospital's goals, financial abilities, marketplace, and other issues. Hospitals must develop these plans independently and use them as the basis for all contracting situations that may arise. As discussed, the essential elements of this plan are:

- Clear statement of goals and objectives
- Financial analysis and forecasting
- Current and future organization and structural arrangements
- Market analysis and projections
- Short-term and long-term projections of patient-base migration
- Analysis of purchaser source-specific cost-to-charge ratio
- Evaluation of competition
- Plans for specific targets in product development, marketing, and contracting

Chapter 3

Understanding Legal Issues

This chapter was written by Mary Layne Ahern, J.D.

Introduction

The legal issues facing a hospital when it considers contracting with an HMO, PPO, or employer vary both in complexity and intensity. Such contractual arrangements may potentially affect all aspects of service delivery, including professional practice, and therefore must be clearly understood and expressly accepted by the contracting parties.

Certain issues involved in a contractual relationship are quite straightforward issues of business law and generally may be handled by in-house counsel. Other legal matters, such as compliance with antitrust laws, may require close scrutiny and expert outside legal advice. Thus, a hospital must consult legal counsel during the negotiation process and before entering into any contractual arrangement in order to sort out the issues.

This chapter sets forth the major legal considerations in the contracting process. It may be used as an advisory legal checklist of sorts, with the proviso that hospital contractual relationships are at issue, not other types of arrangements, such as an incorporated joint venture, that may call for expert legal advice on such subjects as the implications of compliance with tax law or securities law requirements. The starting point must be that a hospital investigates and thoroughly knows the party with whom it is contracting, be it an HMO, PPO, or an individual employer. Many potential legal problems are averted if the hospital has done a careful analysis of the other party's qualifications and goals. Legal absolutes are few, and a hospital should not consider any terms or provisions in the contractual arrangement to be nonnegotiable. Generally, a contract can be arrived at that reflects the particular needs and understandings of the parties.

Ideally, hospital counsel should be present during the management decision-making process concerning the efficacy of entering into a contract for services. Counsel will then be able to structure and word the contract appropriately.

Contractual Elements

This section identifies certain points in a contractual agreement between a hospital and a particular contractor that require special highlighting because of their legal implications. Throughout this section, the word *contractor,* rather than payer, is used to identify the other party to the contract inasmuch as a preferred provider organization (PPO) may not be categorized as a payer.

The following important contract provisions are discussed in this section: responsibilities of hospital and contractor, payment arrangements, confidentiality and medical records, utilization review, dispute resolution, insurance and indemnification, and generic contract terms.

Responsibilities

Contracts include sections on the responsibilities of the parties to the agreement. Such provisions may be quite detailed or general, depending on the parties' choices regarding specific points, although the contract should be reasonably specific regarding the limits of the various responsibilities.

The clarity and precision of the language used to describe the responsibilities of the parties is a most important starting point. Discussions of these sections among the parties often raise or magnify differences of perception and expectation that can be fatal to the success of the contractual arrangement.

Hospital's Responsibilities

Key provisions here focus on the extent of covered services. A hospital's interests are best served by defining the services that its staff and facilities are capable of delivering. In addition, the contract should define services that are not generally covered and the handling of necessary arrangements, either through referrals or by in-hospital special programs for specialty-only care or other specific service offerings. Such a list of covered and noncovered services is generally attached as an exhibit to the body of the contract. Special definitions may be necessary: for example, the contract may specifically detail how out-of-service-area arrangements are to be handled under an HMO agreement or what particular procedures for handling outside laboratory or other tests must be followed.

Contract provisions usually include general language regarding the quality of care. Generally, the hospital agrees that the standards for delivering covered services to eligible persons shall be the same as the standards for delivering care to other patients in the hospital. The contract language must be carefully chosen to avoid violating the hospital's standards of care. A hospital must accept a general responsibility to maintain necessary accreditation, licenses, and insurance. In addition, the contract should include a provision in which the hospital agrees to notify the other party should any material changes in its status occur and should make available necessary and appropriate financial information (see chapter 1).

Contractor's Responsibilities

A contract should include an express provision of the contractor's agreement to pay promptly for services rendered. It should also refer to a contract attachment that describes the rates for services. In addition, the contractor is responsible for obtaining necessary insurance and reinsurance. It must also agree to make available appropriate financial statements, just as the hospital must be prepared to do. Specific provisions dealing with contingencies should the contractor become insolvent are important, especially in a new operation, such as a start-up PPO. In cases of insolvency, for example, current patients must still be cared for and outstanding payments must still be collected. Although an HMO may not appear to be in jeopardy on this point because it is regulated by state and federal law as to reserves, a hospital will nonetheless want to have specific agreements as to the HMO's responsibilities in the event of insolvency.

The contractor must keep complete records regarding the benefits to which the subscriber is entitled. The establishment of and agreement on a mechanism to verify eligibility is important. The contractor is responsible for establishing appropriate procedures for conclusive verification of subscriber eligibility, including, but not limited to, methods to promptly handle errors or changes in eligibility status. Also included in the contractor's responsibilities is the indemnification of the hospital for fraud perpetrated by a subscriber and for any liability exposure of the hospital caused by a subscriber's misunderstanding or misinformation regarding the extent of benefits. The hospital should require that the contractor provide a sample copy of its subscriber agreement.

Marketing plans are also the responsibility of the contractor. Because various promotional methods may be used, the hospital should obtain the right to review and approve any promotional campaign material in which its name is used. An agreement to protect the hospital's name and reputation is appropriate. In addition, the hospital will want to receive a list of other providers participating in a contractual agreement with the contractor.

Finally, the contractor, like the hospital, has the responsibility for maintaining any applicable licenses and insurance and for filing any necessary government-mandated documentation. The contract should also include an agreement that the contractor will comply with applicable laws and regulations and will verify this compliance.

Payment by Contractor and Beneficiary

The contract section regarding payment must contain information on method, timing, and arrangements for appropriate beneficiary payment. The method for computing payment should be carefully negotiated, and including in the contract the option to renegotiate annually both the method and the amounts of payment may be desirable. The complexity of available payment strategies may make these negotiations equally complex.

The contract should include information on the claim form and should specify the requirements for claim submission. Information on payment time periods and claims assignment procedures should also be included in the contract.

The hospital should require the contractor to provide verification that subscribers understand payment arrangements and will abide by them. Such verification is especially important when the hospital must engage in coordination-of-benefits procedures on behalf of the beneficiary. The provisions relating to payment by the contractor's subscribers or employees must be carefully negotiated and structured, including the copayment and deductible arrangements, if any. In addition, the hospital should ensure that it retains the right to seek payment as appropriate directly from the subscribers for noncovered services. The contract should be specific as to the contractor's responsibilities regarding the subscriber's knowledge and understanding of the definition of "any other sources" of payment, the procedures involved in determining the primary and secondary sources, and arrangements for handling combinations of benefits.

Payment methodology and discussion of covered services are affected by arrangements made between the contractor and physicians.

The extent of inclusion or exclusion of physician services from payment rates to hospitals must be clear.

The hospital should be knowledgeable about the payment rates and discounts that physicians have negotiated with certain contractors and about any incentives offered for efficiency. In addition, as discussed later in this chapter, specific concerns regarding hospital-based physicians and the internal contracts governing such arrangements must be addressed.

Confidentiality and Medical Records

Access to certain patient information and documentation is necessary for the operation of a successful utilization review program. The hospital should ensure that plan members are appropriately informed through admission and authorization procedures as to the nature and extent of such information sharing. The contract should state that the utilization control plan will protect confidentiality. It should also state that the contractor is responsible for obtaining authorization from each subscriber for access to such data from the medical record as necessary to conduct the utilization management program and shall provide such authorization to the hospital.

An explicit contractual agreement that each party will abide by applicable laws regarding the confidentiality of medical records is important, as discussed in the section on liability later in this chapter. Also, the circumstances under which information may be released and who will obtain any needed release from the patient must be addressed. The parties must determine the state law requirements regarding patient authorization for release of records before anyone outside of the hospital is allowed to review such records. In addition, the contract should include an explicit provision requiring indemnification of the hospital for potential liability exposure if patient information is improperly or negligently released by the contractor.

Utilization Review

Because careful structuring of the utilization review (UR) plan is of paramount importance, the contract should reflect agreement on the following issues:

- Responsibility for review function: for example, is the hospital or an independent agency responsible for reviews?
- Types of review to be included: for example, are preadmission, admission, concurrent, or retrospective or some combination to be conducted? The contract should include a definition of what is to be reviewed in each type of review.
- Responsibility for costs of review: for example, are the costs of reviews shared by contractor and hospital or borne by the hospital alone?

Generally, the hospital will want to play a major role in the review process either by taking it on itself or at least by providing strong input in alliance with physicians.

Specifics of UR procedures should be defined in an attachment to the agreement. Such specifics include credentials of reviewers, appropriate communication and verification mechanisms regarding use of services, and especially, confirmation of the fact that a pre-admission or concurrent UR determination is advisory to the health care provider and does not constitute a treatment decision. Defined standards of medical necessity and emergency care are important to this process, as are defined criteria used by reviewers for recommendations.

Noncovered or Disallowed Services, Appeal Process, and Dispute Resolution

The contract must include procedures for handling payment when the service was given pursuant to the patient's request and the physician's order but was not covered or when the entity responsible for utilization review recommends that payment not be made (a related discussion of this issue appears in a section on fair dealing later in this chapter). A clear appeals process that covers all types of payment denials, either preadmission, concurrent, or retroactive, must be included in the contract.

Mechanisms for the resolution of disputes should be a separate contract provision. Such mechanisms may include arbitration procedures, including conferences. The hospital should insist on methods short of litigation to attempt the resolution of problems between itself and the contractors. Although dispute resolution is dealt with in statutes regarding health maintenance organizations (HMOs), it may be negotiated when contracting with an employer or a preferred provider organization (PPO).

The hospital should ensure that the contractor and subscribers agree on a grievance procedure for handling complaints. Also, the contract should specify how any breaches of the various contract provisions will be handled.

Insurance and Indemnification

As discussed in the section "Liability Issues" later in this chapter, both parties to the contract must obtain and maintain adequate levels of insurance for professional and financial liability. Indemnification, or hold-harmless, clauses should be carefully scrutinized; and if they are included, the hospital must insist that they apply to both parties. In any case, counsel should be consulted regarding the effect of such a provision on current liability policies and under state law. In addition, the contract should specify that the contractor will require each contracted provider (physician or hospital) to carry a specified amount of insurance. Also, the contractor and the hospital shall promptly agree to inform the other of any legal action arising out of services provided to subscribers by the hospital.

Generic Contract Terms

Finally, all contracts should contain the following provisions:

- The term of the contract and any desired automatic renewal clauses.
- Termination circumstances that may trigger the end of the contractual arrangement, including reasonable standards when "for cause"; automatic provisions regarding license loss or other illegalities that may jeopardize subscriber welfare; and a force majeure ("Act of God") provision in case of natural disasters. Also included should be an agreement as to the care of patients in the hospital at the time of termination and arrangements for payment under these circumstances.
- Times and methods for renegotiation of contract terms, especially payment rates.

HMO Laws and Regulations

The hospital should be thoroughly familiar with the provisions and requirements in state and federal laws and regulations that apply to HMOs and competitive medical plans (CMPs). As a responsible and cautious party to an agreement, a hospital entering into a contractual arrangement with a federally qualified HMO or federally certified CMP should review the basic requirements of the laws and regulations and should be satisfied that its contractual partner is in compliance. The requirements include:

- Professional liability coverage
- Insolvency insurance and the approach used for protection of members from charges that may result from HMO insolvency
- Reserves, as stipulated by state law
- Certain minimum basic benefits
- Subscriber-related requirements, including a limitation on the percentage of subscribers from a specialized population
- Mandate that the governing board of the HMO be one-third subscribers

Because state HMO laws and regulations vary, they must be closely examined by a hospital before it enters into a contract with an HMO. The HMO's corporate status, that is, its for-profit or not-for-profit status, and requirements for conversion from one status to another are important to a hospital's complete examination of a potential arrangement with an HMO. Each state's laws and regulations include mandated benefits and requirements for bonds and reserves.

PPO Laws and Insurance Regulations

A hospital contracting with a PPO must be thoroughly familiar with the legal and regulatory environment relating to the contractor and with the specific contractor's structure and status. The following characteristics are probably the only ones common to all PPOs:

- A PPO is a managed care system characterized by the provision of incentives in the form of discounts or penalties to consumer-subscribers to use certain preselected preferred providers.

- A PPO contracts with selected physicians, hospitals, and perhaps, other facilities or providers to make up a panel of preferred providers but does not assume indemnification risks for subscribers' covered services.

Beyond these basics, PPOs may take many organizational forms, such as independent corporations, corporations formed by hospital holding companies, or partnerships between physicians and hospitals. Each of these structures has different inherent legal considerations. However, for the purposes of this book, the hospital interested in entering into a straightforward contractual relationship with a PPO needs to be concerned with the PPO's compliance with statutory and regulatory mandates and the PPO's financial, marketing, and administrative strengths.

Four categories of laws affect PPOs: insurance, health service plan, HMO legislation, and specific PPO legislation. Many states have enacted laws specifically regulating the formation and operation of PPOs. Generally, these laws remove certain barriers to PPO formation and also may regulate PPO operation, including aspects of contracting. A hospital considering a contractual relationship with a PPO must be thoroughly familiar with any existing legislation in its state. In addition, PPO statutes generally modify regulatory provisions found in insurance laws. Such modifications may be found in freedom-of-choice guarantees for subscribers and limits on benefit design and policy premiums to curb unfair discrimination against beneficiaries.

When no specific statute regarding PPOs exists, a hospital considering a contractual relationship with a PPO must study the statutory and legal environment concerning other relevant laws in its state. Depending on their sponsors, structures, and services, some PPOs may be considered a type of third-party contractor that may be subject to regulations on a state-by-state basis under state insurance; health service plans, which are generally defined as entities that contract with providers to provide services to subscribers and assume the risk for illness; or HMO laws and regulations. If a PPO's structure makes it subject to these regulations, it may be required to comply with subscriber freedom of choice and various other rules. Many PPOs do not fall into these regulated categories, but a hospital considering a contractual relationship must be familiar with the possible impact of applicable laws and regulations.

As far as operational provisions are concerned, PPO statutes may cover the following issues:

- *Exclusive provider organization (EPO).* Some states directly prohibit the establishment of PPOs that prevent subscribers from obtaining reimbursement for services received from other than a preferred provider. Others allow EPOs but regulate them, usually in terms of minimum benefits, standards for availability of services, and independent review requirements.
- *Provider participation.* Some statutes require that the PPO include on its panel any provider willing to meet the terms and conditions set by the PPO. Generally, such provisions contain, in addition, a prohibition against *unreasonable discrimination* among providers in the terms and conditions outlined.
- *Antitrust exemption.* Contract negotiations with a PPO may, in some states, be declared exempt from the state antitrust laws. However, this exemption does not apply to federal antitrust statutes.

If a PPO meets the definitional criteria of an insurance company under state law, such as assuming any of the economic risk associated with specific contingencies, it is subject to certain mandated requirements. These requirements may include maintenance of capital reserves, the insured's freedom of choice of providers, and provisions that prohibit unfair discrimination among subscribers. In addition, a PPO may meet the definition of an insurance agent or broker if it handles or negotiates applications on behalf of insurers. Also, some states regulate the third parties that administer insurance benefits for others, and a PPO may possibly fall within the definition of such an administrator.

Health service plans, which are regulated in all states, have detailed requirements regarding corporate status and administrative procedures. If a PPO is so structured that it falls within the health service plan definition, it must meet at least these two requirements: freedom of choice of providers for subscribers and allowance of all licensed providers to participate.

Finally, depending on the chosen structure and method of arranging for services, a PPO may be subject to regulation as an HMO.

As noted in the previous section on HMOs, HMO regulation varies from state to state.

Liability Issues

The following sections briefly discuss the various liability issues that must be considered before a hospital enters into a contractual relationship: malpractice, confidentiality, fair dealing, and referrals. The structure of the utilization management plan and the selection of providers are the main sources of liability concerns.

Malpractice

Malpractice liability is a primary issue in contractual arrangements. The hospital's duty to protect its patients from negligent acts is not altered by a contractual arrangement. The duty to carefully select staff and the responsibility for the acts of its employees and agents, such as independent physicians with privileges to practice at that hospital, do not become less important.

An HMO or a PPO must conduct its operations, especially the operation of the UR program, in a nonnegligent manner. According to recent legal trends, the HMO or PPO may be liable for the negligent denial or withholding of authorization for a medical procedure. Also, the HMO or PPO, as the utilization review agent, may be liable for authorizing premature discharge. However, the hospital's duty of care is probably not mitigated by the HMO's or PPO's action, and therefore the hospital could be liable for malpractice as well. For this reason, the hospital may wish to insist on some mechanism that would involve member-patients in authorization procedures regarding payment for medical treatment, at least to the extent of ensuring full information on the reasons for any utilization-control decision.

The so-called corporate negligence theory that makes a hospital liable for independent physicians as part of the duty of care it must exercise in selecting physicians may be extended in the case of a hospital-PPO or hospital-HMO contract. A hospital may be held to a higher review standard because of the multiple relationships involved in contracting with an HMO or a PPO. For example, a hospital that takes an active part in selecting physicians for the PPO or sponsors the PPO itself may be subject to a higher standard of care than one that only contracted with the PPO.

Confidentiality

Privacy and confidentiality of medical information are other issues of potential liability. State statutes protect medical information, and federal regulations concerning treatment of alcohol and drug abuse and mental illness contain additional confidentiality protections.

Disclosure of information for any reason must be preceded by patient consent except when professionally related determinations, such as use of the information in a medical staff peer review committee, are involved. To the extent specified in each state's law, these committee records are protected, and therefore disclosure for such purposes generally will not jeopardize the patient's rights. All important protections must be explicitly agreed to in the contract.

Fair Dealing

Other liability concerns are of greater importance to the physician's relationship with an HMO or a PPO than with the hospital's. If a provider recommends a medical procedure and the HMO-sponsored or PPO-sponsored review program recommends that the procedure not be authorized, the provider may claim interference with patient relationships. In addition, courts recognize an implied covenant of good faith and fair dealing, and member-patients may sue if they do not receive the benefits to which they believe they are entitled.

Referrals

Any negligent interference with the patient's right to reasonable continuity of care and concomitant referral arrangements may give rise to liability. Referral arrangements must be made with due care; and if the HMO or PPO has specific panels of physicians and surgeons under contract for specialty care, it must exercise care in the selection of those panels. However, the hospital may not be absolved from liability from negligent referrals for further care.

The best solution for the hospital is to insist that membership agreements include sufficient disclosure of arrangements. In these cases, as in all situations touching on liability insurance, the hospital's insurance carrier should review the contracts to determine any effect on coverage.

Antitrust Issues

Probably the most frequently raised legal concern in hospital contractual relationships is the possibility of violating antitrust laws. Generally, potential antitrust exposure is most likely to be in the areas of prohibition against unreasonable restraint of trade and actual or attempted monopolization, as described in the Sherman Act (15 U.S.C. §§ 1 *et seq.*).

The Sherman Act prohibits "contracts, combinations or conspiracies" made in restraint of trade. To violate the first section of this law, two or more separate entities must have entered into a contract that results in unreasonable restraint of competition. In addition, the second section prohibits monopolizing activities. Other laws relating to antitrust are the Federal Trade Commission Act (15 U.S.C. § 45), which prohibits unfair methods of competition and unfair or deceptive acts or practices, and the Clayton Act (15 U.S.C. §§ 13-14, 18), which prohibits price discrimination, certain exclusive dealing, tying contracts, and certain mergers and acquisitions.

Any analysis of possible antitrust problems should be made on a case-by-case basis. Such an analysis is a fact-intensive scrutiny that includes close looks at the parties involved, the market, the specific purpose of the arrangement, and its effects on competition. Although legitimate contractual arrangements have the potential for increasing economic efficiency or capacity—prime reasons that allow a venture to avoid violation of antitrust laws—they will be scrutinized closely; and as a result, the need for legal advice in this area is paramount. Although the procompetitive effects of certain contractual relationships may be significant, others may be automatically considered to violate antitrust laws because of their anticompetitive effects.

Because certain violations are considered to be extreme in their anticompetitive effects, public injury resulting from such contracts is presumed, and no examination of markets or other factors is made by the court. The so-called per se violations of particular relevance to this discussion of contractual arrangements are price fixing and group boycotts or exclusive dealings.

Price fixing

Price fixing, which is a violation of antitrust laws, occurs when competitors agree to charge uniform prices or give uniform discounts; in other words, price fixing is collusive conduct that sets prices, for example, minimum or maximum fees or discounts. Such agreements among competitors (horizontal agreements) that have the effect of suppressing competition are per se illegal, and the courts do not consider justifications for the agreement. However, if the contracts are between buyers and sellers (vertical agreements) to establish prices or discounts, such agreements are generally analyzed under the less stringent *rule-of-reason* standard, and the courts test the procompetitive versus anticompetitive effects of the contracts. What the courts look for is the promotion of competition; and in doing so, the courts examine the purpose and effect of the agreements to determine if restraint of competition exists, what the market power of each of the participants to the agreement is, and if legitimate business purposes can be achieved by other less restrictive means.

For example, PPO arrangements are generally analyzed under the rule-of-reason standard. In an arrangement between hospitals and other providers and a nonprovider-controlled PPO, price-fixing concerns may be minimized if the contracting process is done on an individual basis. If no unlawful horizontal conduct has taken place, that is, if competing providers have not discussed and negotiated a collective fee-setting or discount arrangement, contracts between one buyer (the PPO) and many sellers (hospital and physician providers) are not viewed as illegal price-fixing violations of antitrust laws.

If the PPO itself is provider sponsored, its contractual arrangements may be more carefully analyzed. Generally, however, the agreements probably still are analyzed under the rule-of-reason standard instead of being declared unlawful per se as price fixing. The reason for such treatment is that the price setting is ancillary to the main purpose of the arrangement, which is to enhance competition through the creation of the PPO. However, courts may place greater emphasis on analyzing market power and generally may take a closer rule-of-reason look at such arrangements.

Exclusive Dealing

Certain conditions of a hospital's participation in a contractual agreement, such as requiring full medical staff approval of the hospital-

HMO contract, may be considered to be in restraint of trade. Another type of violation, one that requires a lesser degree of scrutiny, is an *unlawful boycott or exclusive dealing arrangement.* To determine whether a contract will be deemed exclusive dealing and therefore in violation of antitrust laws, an analysis is undertaken to determine what percentage of the market (however defined) is tied up by the arrangement and whether competitors entering the market are significantly hampered. Courts may use a *qualitative test,* which involves weighing procompetitive reasons against actual anticompetitive effects, or a *quantitative test,* which looks at the degree of market restraint and the time length of such restraint.

If, for example, a PPO and selected providers enter into a contract that excludes a hospital or physician and clearly intends to limit competition, such an agreement is considered a per se violation of antitrust laws. However, if the parties to the arrangement did not contract with the intent to limit competition, then the courts will apply the less strict rule-of-reason standard when analyzing the contract. Courts generally will acknowledge the advancement of consumer interests in the efficiencies created as well as the group's economic interests.

To prove that a contractual arrangement between a PPO and its chosen providers violates antitrust laws as an unlawful refusal to deal, an excluded hospital's argument generally may hinge on whether or not it is deprived of essential business relationships by such an arrangement. The analysis of this allegation includes an inquiry examining the PPO's percentage of the market to determine if it has undue market power and an examination of the purpose and effect of the alleged monopolization.

The analysis of any contractual arrangement for unlawful monopolization and exclusive dealing must be carried out separately for each party to the contract, with each market examined and intent scrutinized. In all cases, antitrust compliance concerns are sensitive issues and must receive careful, expert legal analysis, but such concerns should not be barriers to legitimate cooperative contractual arrangements.

Hospital-Physician Relationships

Certain provisions regarding physicians should be included in contracts with PPOs and HMOs. The hospital should clearly state the role that its internal physician organization will play and the fact that its responsibilities do not include a duty to accept any particular physician as a member of its medical staff. Because the hospital is ultimately responsible for the selection of its medical staff, it must retain its independence regarding choices of physicians. In addition, a provision specifying that no member of the hospital medical staff may be forced to accept particular patients may be appropriate. Other issues affecting physicians have been discussed earlier in this chapter where appropriate.

Conclusion

The legal issues discussed in this chapter are intended to highlight important aspects of the contract between a hospital and an HMO, PPO, or employer and to provide important background considerations for the negotiation process. Although certain law-related matters may be handled best by in-house counsel and others by outside specialists, the key point is that legal counsel must be consulted during the negotiation and contracting processes. Legal counsel can provide guidance as to the particular terms and provisions that require detailed attention and can direct the process so that the hospital client's particular strategic goals are met. The hospital should never consider any terms or contractual provisions to be nonnegotiable but should consult with legal counsel to negotiate any modifications, additions, or deletions that are deemed necessary.

Part II

Planning Strategies for Contracting

Chapter 4

Implementing Direct Employer Contracts

Introduction

As used in this chapter, *direct employer contracting* is defined as direct contractual relationships between health care providers and employers as purchasers of services. The purpose of these arrangements is to promote flexible, direct contracting without the inclusion of such middlemen as insurers and preferred provider organizations (PPOs). Many employers now believe that significant advantages can be achieved through developing and controlling their own arrangements and working directly with health care providers.

Direct contracting between health care providers and employers is an innovative method for combining the resources, goals, and methodologies of health care providers and consumers of health care services to achieve the common objectives of high-quality services, cost-effectiveness, and market control. This potentially cooperative arrangement is accomplished by working with individual large employers, which are either nationally dispersed or regionally centralized, or through multiple employer approaches, including coalitions and trade associations. Contractual relationships developed between purchasers and providers of health care services can represent a cooperative approach to solving health care cost and management problems. These approaches are being used in the states of California, Colorado, and Georgia, among others. The approach eliminates the direct role of an insurer or separate PPO legal entity.

Clearly, several advantages exist for hospitals involved in direct contractual relationships. If properly structured, these relationships provide hospitals with a direct and controlled relationship with a defined organization of service utilizers to which they can market their health care services. The hospital no longer has to market directly to several different purchasing organizations or insurers; rather, a controlled group of users (the employer's own employees) are directly accessible to the hospital. This arrangement permits the hospital to implement creative direct-marketing approaches that are potentially more effective in getting patients for the hospital. Further, in this kind of arrangement, the exchange of utilization and cost information is easier to manage and more useful.

However, direct contracting may also have some administrative complications for hospitals. Multiple contracts, reporting requirements, and legal review of contracting issues can become burdensome as contracting increases. The benefits of potential contracts, such as volume and market exposure, must be weighed against administrative requirements. Further, through the negotiation process, every effort should be made to streamline the arrangements as much as possible. If, as in a recently implemented program, a group of employers work together on project development but contract separately, contract provisions should be standardized to the extent possible within legal constraints.

Employers that become involved in this type of contractual relationship gain several advantages. They have direct control over where their employees seek care, how that care is paid for, and how the contracting provider's services are being marketed to employees. Employers can directly design flexible benefits plans that encourage employees to seek services from contract providers. Further, the employers benefit from direct information exchange and from these cooperative types of long-term working relationships. However, administrative requirements for the employer may be increased as these arrangements are developed. More direct responsibility is required, and this responsibility translates to more staff and administrative time required on the part of the employer.

A hospital seeking to become involved in direct contractual relationships should have included this goal as part of its overall strategic plan. The plan should include a definition of goals and objectives, an assessment of the hospital's internal capacity to take on the added administrative duties required in such arrangements, a description of the market potential for direct contractual relationships, and information on which companies can provide an appropriately sized market for the hospital and which industries should be targeted. Further, the strategic plan should include a method for evaluating potential arrangements and forecasting outcomes and a method for evaluating each contract in terms of administrative requirements, profitability, quality assurance, utilization management, and market potential.

Contracting Team

The team of professionals charged with facilitating the hospital's direct contracting should include a contract manager, a person involved in the financial management of the hospital, a marketing expert familiar with the local market, and legal counsel. The general responsibilities of this primary team are evaluating and negotiating the contracts, determining the legal issues involved, and monitoring their long-term effects. The specific responsibilities of each member of the primary contracting team are as follows:

- *Contract manager.* The hospital's contract manager should be responsible for all administrative tasks required in responding to proposals and in contracting and negotiating with all purchasers of health care services, who may be employers, PPOs, health maintenance organizations (HMOs), commercial insurers, or others. This responsibility includes the development of background information on the purchaser, coordination of the team schedules, coordination of proposal development, administration of contracts, and any required coordination with physician groups. The contract manager should also assist in employee communication and in the development of marketing materials for the program. In short, the contract manager has coordinating and administrative responsibility for the entire contracting process. The level of decision-making responsibility delegated to the contract manager depends on what other staff is available. Some contract managers have senior positions; others are middle managers. The decision to hire a separate contract manager or use other staff depends on the amount of contracting undertaken by a hospital and the availability of appropriate staff members.
- *Financial specialist.* The financial specialist, or possibly the hospital's chief financial officer (CFO), evaluates internal costs, including contract administration costs and service costs related to pricing. This person is also responsible for the evaluation and development of competitive payment mechanisms and rates that are appropriate for the specific contract and advantageous to the hospital. These mechanisms may include risk arrangements (discussed in chapter 2), incentive pools, or volume-related payment mechanisms. Familiarity with pricing techniques and risk evaluation is required.
- *Marketing expert.* A marketing expert provides the team with knowledge of the hospital's market base and an understanding

of the potential contractors' market power and influence. This team member also develops marketing strategies based on the demographics of the market area and the specific demographics of the interested employer. The market expert should also be familiar with the competitive situation within the marketplace and its effects on the contracting relationship. This person also develops any new marketing materials that may be required and is responsible for employee communication efforts, including presentations, material development, and other creative efforts. The marketing expert is further responsible for developing a marketing strategy for each market segment. Frequently, this position is combined with that of the contract manager.

• *Legal counsel.* Legal counsel is required in contractual relationship situations. The health care attorney's role is to review contracting documents and ascertain any legal problems that may be encountered.

Other members of a contracting team include the hospital chief executive officer (CEO) and the utilization review (UR) manager. Their services are required on an as-needed basis and primarily for the negotiation process. The UR manager or coordinator is responsible for internal UR and interfacing with external UR requirements. Because UR is a key negotiation issue, a knowledgeable person must be available throughout the negotiation process to answer questions, verify services, and review proposed plans or contract issues. The hospital CEO may be required as an addition to the team in situations in which the importance of the purchaser to the hospital demands a high-level negotiator.

Another ad hoc member of the management team is the hospital's data manager. Data systems requirements are generally discussed by the employer and the hospital during negotiations. Administrative interface with the employer's external claims administrator or the employer's own self-administration system is a key area in negotiations. A qualified systems expert who is currently working with the hospital's internal data systems may be required for technical aspects of contract discussions.

Many hospitals do not have the resources for allocating so many staff members to the contracting process. If necessary, responsibilities can be handled by a smaller staff, especially at the onset of activities. Many of the tasks can be undertaken by hospital CEOs and CFOs. However, the impact of taking these executive staff members' time away from their regular management roles should be considered when developing contracting plans.

The contracting team is responsible for the general evaluation of each contract prior to introducing it into the hospital's review and approval process. The general issues that need to be evaluated are:

- Level of hospital financial liability
- Level of risk being shared or undertaken by the hospital; potential loss or profitability for the hospital
- Potential market share increase or retention represented by the contract
- Potential market impact if the hospital does not contract
- Power of the individual employer or the industry in which it operates
- Utilization management implications of the contract and cost of administration
- Quality of care issues arising from contract stipulations

These general issues are the key to the overall success of a contracting arrangement between employers and hospital providers. All of them must also be taken into account in identifying the potential pitfalls of *not* contracting.

Marketing Issues

Generally, direct contracting is initiated by employers, and hospitals are often placed in a reactive rather than a proactive marketing role. Nevertheless, before becoming involved in any direct contractual relationship, the hospital should develop a thorough marketing plan. The development of this plan includes examining, on a broad basis, all of the strategic issues outlined in part I of this book. A market survey, as described in chapter 2, is required for the development of the marketing plan.

Market segmentation and product differentiation are especially important aspects of a marketing plan. The hospital's markets should be segmented by industry type; insurance arrangements of purchasers (that is, fully insured, minimum premium, self-insured); and purchaser size by number of employees and by the type of product that is likely to be purchased. The evaluation of each market segment should take into consideration each of the hospital's product lines and the applicability of the product line to the market segments. For example, a middle-size, self-insured or partially self-insured employer may be developing cost-management programs. This employer may be interested in implementing cost-management programs other than the comprehensive PPO products available from the hospital. These products may include chemical dependency programs, wellness programs, worker's compensation programs, or other types of programs less comprehensive than a full-service provider contractual arrangement. The hospital would need to be able to segment its products into programs that would appeal to this employer.

In developing strategies to meet the needs of each targeted market segment or employer, the hospital should define individual products that can be made available independently. A minimum goal is to "get a foot in the door" with an employer, if only to distribute a hospital brochure or participate in a wellness or an employee education program. This strategy may lead to a full-service contract in the second or third year. Other strategies for reaching different market segments may include provision of certain types of utilization and cost data, guarantees on prices or savings, or specialty-service contracts for open-heart surgery or other types of services.

Another important aspect of the marketing plan is forecasting. Forecasting allows a hospital to determine the level of focus and the manpower and resources to be allocated to the effort. It can also help to determine the feasibility of direct contracting with employers. For example, direct contracting may not be as feasible in rural areas as it is in urban areas because rural areas generally have few large-size or medium-size employers.

In determining the feasibility of direct approaches to marketing hospital services, the assigned hospital staff should develop historical background information specific to employers and coalition efforts in the community. Sources of information include listings of employers produced by local chambers of commerce and by the U.S. Chamber of Commerce and trade association listings of coalitions. These lists are available in most public libraries. These sources give company names, number of employees, and other basic information on the industry in which the company is involved. The *Directory of Health Care Coalitions in the United States,* published by the American Hospital Association, not only lists general information about the members but also includes information on the individual and collective activities of the coalition. Other sources of information may be available on a state-by-state basis from state hospital associations, state and regional chambers of commerce, and other sources in each state.

Further market information should be developed on employers currently using hospital services. This information, collected through the hospital's data system, includes total dollars as well as days and number of admissions. Data for the current year and trends over the previous one to three years are necessary. Employers accountable for the higher volume levels obviously are primary targets in considering market retention through direct contracting arrangements. However, they also pose a more significant power base in their negotiations with the hospital because they represent a sizable segment of the hospital's business. Generally, an employer with 2 percent to 5 percent of total patient days during a 12-month period is in a favorable negotiating position.

Additional information required for market feasibility is an assessment of the competition within the marketplace. This assessment includes other individual hospitals; managed care plans, including PPOs and health maintenance organizations (HMOs); and any other organization that offers the same services to purchasers that the hospital does. Evaluation of the hospital's current role within these organizations as well as the competitive impact if the hospital is a nonmember is important to this assessment. An analysis of services, financial statistics, pricing, reputation, and geographic location is also important.

Ascertaining staffing needs for the contracting process and for any type of marketing efforts that may be required is also a part of the analysis. Further, the development of a marketing budget and the forecasting of sales and time frames is an integral part of the process. Actuarial projections of utilization patterns for the group covered by the terms of a contract or for the general population in the area help determine the level of risk being assumed by the hospital and the suitability of the direct contracting approach for the market area.

Marketing strategies required for direct contracting include direct one-on-one marketing efforts and the use of community contacts as a resource. These efforts may include marketing informally to board members and potential board members from the employer community or through other community relations programs the hospital has generated. The hospital should keep in close touch with employer coalitions and participate in their educational and other programs as a means of monitoring the philosophies and health care program activities of employers in the area.

Financial Planning Issues

A hospital considering direct contracting with an employer or group of employers must be able to predict the financial impact of the proposed contract. This process includes estimating the cost of fulfilling the contract terms and the potential for revenue generation, both direct and indirect.

Before examining these basic issues, a hospital should determine its financial goals for entering into the relationship. In pricing health care services under a contract, the hospital must decide whether its goals are specifically to increase profits, retain threatened market share, break even, or attain a combination of these goals. Overall decisions depend on the complexity of the marketplace, the hospital's and purchaser's sophistication in contracting, and the competitive forces facing the hospital both currently and in the near future.

Using the information developed within the strategic marketing plan, a hospital should be able to project sales and revenue for defined time frames, such as for one year and three years. Projections of revenue flow can be made by means of a combined review of hospital cost experience and actuarial analysis of the employer's employee population.

The major revenue source, which requires in-depth examination, is patient revenue from the provision of medical services. These revenues accumulate in accordance with the negotiated rates and fee schedules contained in the contract with the employer. The services, which are provided directly by the hospital, may include inpatient and outpatient services and other programs, such as chemical dependency or mental health services, that are organized and operated through the hospital.

Direct administrative revenue may accrue from employer contracts based on administrative services other than inpatient services provided directly by the hospital. These services may include spin-off products such as utilization management programs; referral services for which a charge can be assessed; a hot-line service; or development of employee communication or other programs for which the hospital charges a fee. Generally, in a direct employer contract, these services are a minor source of revenue. Most of them are included in the overall general hospital services contract and are not billed separately.

Another element to be measured in contracting is the cost of administering the contract. Precise cost determinations must be made for each activity or service required, including utilization management, administrative procedures such as verification of benefits and billing, and marketing efforts. All fixed and variable costs should be analyzed and weighed against the potential revenue outcome of the contract.

The effect of capital requirements on pricing of services is also an important consideration in contracting. If the hospital is, or will be, involved in capital-intensive projects, it may not be able to price its services as competitively as other hospitals in the community do. Less competitive prices are not always a complete negative to purchasers, but they do require specialized marketing approaches or creative pricing methodologies. A thorough explanation of projects, current or planned, and their value to the purchaser is important. For example, a hospital negotiating an employer contract on the West Coast had recently completed a major building project that had the effect of bringing its ratio of long-term debt to total assets to 59 percent. The employer was aware of this through Medicare cost-report analysis and, because of other negative financial indicators, was concerned about whether the hospital would be able to maintain proposed pricing levels. Negotiations were concluded with prices somewhat higher than initial proposals but with guaranteed three-year increase limitations.

Assessing the impact and the methodology of risk sharing required by a contract is also an important issue for hospitals (risk sharing is discussed in greater detail in chapter 2). If a hospital is contracting on a significant risk-taking basis, be it capitation, global case rates, or any other significant risk arrangement, careful analysis of the impact of that risk should be undertaken by management. Figure 2-3 outlines several payment arrangement options from the perspective of the amount of associated provider risk and the data needed to monitor the effectiveness of the arrangement. A yearly evaluation of total risk represented in all hospital contracts as well as a contract-by-contract analysis is recommended. This evaluation can be completed through actuarial analysis by an outside actuarial firm.

Employers often use actuarial analyses of the associated level of risk and potential-savings outcomes as a part of their provider negotiation strategies. Hospitals should also calculate the level of risk and the potential revenue generation associated with each contract.

An actuarial analysis of potential employer savings includes projections of employee migration to selected providers and the effects of negotiated rates. Actuaries can project savings based on an employer's previous cost experience. Issues such as costs for ancillary and routine services, necessary versus unnecessary admissions, and potential for outpatient surgery are evaluated. Factored into the analysis is the cost of benefits-plan coverage, coordination of benefits, and credits for incentives to use selected providers. Figure 4-1 is an abbreviated example of an actuarial report of projected savings. In this example, incurred costs for two previous years are shown together with projected year-3 costs without negotiated rates. Costs with negotiated rates and varying employee migration levels are noted in the four right-hand columns of the table and estimated savings also are shown.

Risk sharing has become a contracting option that is increasingly attractive to employers. As long as the employer's administrators can manage the payment methods, risk sharing is viewed favorably. Risk sharing encourages employer respect for hospitals' utilization management programs, inasmuch as careful monitoring is in everyone's best interest when all are at financial risk (several risk-sharing arrangements are discussed in chapter 2).

In specifying terms for payment, the hospital's cash flow must be protected. If the contract represents a small volume, the issue is not as crucial as it is with a large employer or coalition of employers. The contract often sets a time limit for payment of outstanding invoices.

All of these financial issues lead to the need for a complete ongoing evaluation of the contract's impact on a hospital's bottom line. This evaluation of data should help weigh the possible gain, loss, or

Figure 4-1. Example of an Actuarial Analysis of Employer Savings

All Hospitals	Year 1 (Incurred)	Year 2 (Incurred)	Year 3 (Projected without Nego- tiated Rates)	Year 3 (Projected with Negotiated Rates at Various Migration Levels)		
				30%	50%	78%	92%
Total hospital costs	$1,611,593	$1,907,935	$1,070,445	$982,335	$968,858	$911,999	$870,061
Total savings				$ 88,110	$101,587	$158,446	$200,384

maintenance of hospital market share along with the profitability of that market share. In the first year, a contract may not be financially advantageous to a hospital, but in the long term, it may prove useful in retaining market share of an industry or in a particular region. When appropriate, the hospital should be flexible enough to allow the idea of retaining market share to outweigh some of the less attractive financial aspects of an agreement. On the basis of financial data, a hospital may choose to cancel an employer contract and seek access to employees through HMOs or other organizations offered by the employer.

Individual employers or groups of employers face financial constraints themselves in contracting with health care providers. They are limited by the administrative abilities of either their external claims administrators or their internal claims processing system. They are also limited by their ability to control employees and assist in achieving goals of containing health care costs. Employers are constrained by the administrative complexity of monitoring data related to the contract and by their own unique employee relations situations. All of these issues affect the level of sophistication with which they negotiate and contract with a hospital.

Organizational Structure

The organizational structures of both the purchaser and the hospital become an issue in direct contracting. Understanding the purchaser's structure and its impact on negotiation issues and hospital administrative costs is important. The hospital's own structure as it affects the negotiations and implementation of the contract is also important from the purchaser's perspective.

Purchaser's Structure

An arrangement in which an employer or group of employers contracts directly with health care providers requires little if any formal organizational structure devoted specifically to this activity. Depending on the goals and objectives of the employer, no formal structure may exist, or contracts may be executed through an employer-sponsored cooperative or multiple-employer trust.

Multiple employers choosing to contract through an organizational structure may do so through an arrangement of employers according to an organizational form known as a *shared health options purchasing (SHOP) plan.* This term refers to an organization in which employers work together to select and purchase health care services. The key to this structure is the vertical integration of services, including all services required by the employers' benefits plans. This vertical integration is achieved by contracting with hospitals that offer all of the varieties of services required or by contracting with other selected provider organizations.

The SHOP plan may take one of two organization structures. Figure 4-2 incorporates a separate legal entity (often a cooperative) that acts through group contracts on behalf of employers A, B, and C. Provider services are obtained through one contract per provider group. This model, which is in operation in several areas of the country, is relatively easy for employers and providers to administer.

Figure 4-3 is a variation of figure 4-2. It incorporates direct individual contracts between each employer and each provider group. Coalition or trade association members have incorporated this model to avoid antitrust implications and to provide for flexibility in benefits plan design, implementation dates, and provider selection. In this figure, each company retains current relationships with their existing claims administrators. The management group assists in provider selection and negotiation and in the ongoing operation of a data base for monitoring the program. The claims administrators provide the management group with data that is analyzed and reported to employers and providers on a regular basis.

A hospital should evaluate the significance of the structure that has been developed by contracting employers to determine the advantages and disadvantages of participation with that organized group. Clearly, working directly with the users of the hospital's service has advantages. However, the administrative aspects of direct, individual contracts can be more complicated than the administrative aspects of group contracts. Multiple contracts can significantly complicate the hospital's administrative process.

Evaluating the administrative capabilities of claims administrators used by contracting employers, individually or collectively, is crucial to the successful functioning of a contract. Employers that are partially or fully self-insured often contract with third-party administrators

Figure 4-2. SHOP Plan

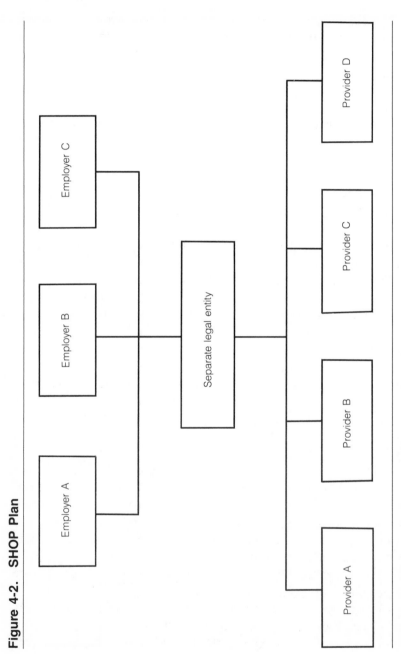

Figure 4-3. Variation on SHOP Plan

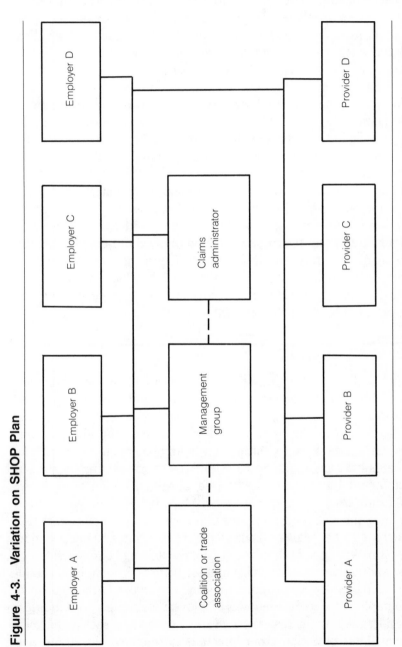

to perform administrative functions required in claims adjudication and payment. Employers may also choose to be self-administered (that is, to perform these functions internally) or enter into a more limited administrative services only arrangement. Large insurers as well as independent organizations may perform these functions under contract.

Problems may arise when claims administrators are unable to coordinate administrative functions required by the contract between the employer and the hospital. For example, an employer's contract with a hospital may incorporate complicated payment arrangements with high levels of risk sharing, utilization management data requirements, and sophisticated incentive pools. If the employer's claims administrator cannot administer the system, the arrangement will not function and administrative snags will be severe. One suggested approach, if the employer is willing, is to meet with the external claims administrator and the employer or group of employers to determine exactly how the relationship will function over the long term. Several employers have been in contract situations in which they have been forced to change the terms of the provider contract or change administrators because of such complications.

Hospital's Structure and Services

A hospital's own organizational structure should be examined for its adaptability to contracting. If the hospital has holding companies and subsidiary corporations, how will those structures affect contracting for services? Must an employer contract with each subsidiary, or may services be contracted for through the holding-company arrangement? What is the easiest and most flexible way of contracting for the services of the hospital and the hospital corporation? These issues are important to contracting employers. Many hospitals have developed separate subsidiary corporations that have the power to contract on behalf of the hospital and a related physician group, and such arrangements may be positively perceived by purchasing companies.

Another aspect of organizational structures that employers evaluate is geographic access to employers and employees. Lack of adequate geographic access often requires employers to contract with multiple providers. A hospital that offers a variety of services, such as an emergency clinic, physician group practices in numerous locations, and other outpatient medical services conveniently available to employees, may have an advantage over competitors in negotiating with an employer. For this reason, many hospitals have developed strategies to acquire or assist in developing group practices and other services in strategic locations.

Medical services that are often most important to a contracting employer include inpatient hospital services, outpatient surgery and other ambulatory care services, home health care, pharmacy services, wellness programs, and organized physician group practices. The employer often looks to the hospital to organize physicians into group practices if no such groups are available as contract partners.

Hospital's Affiliations

Another issue that should be examined is the value of a hospital's participation in provider network organizations. Depending on the sophistication of a purchaser and the administrative capabilities at the individual hospitals, these organizations can prove useful in contracting situations. They can arrange for, negotiate, and monitor all contracts for the hospital. However, some employers may desire to contract directly with the hospitals and not through such marketing organizations. An important consideration for hospitals is to retain flexibility to facilitate appropriate independent employer contracts and long-term cooperative relationships.

In some cases, exclusive arrangements with marketing networks can be detrimental to a hospital. In a recent contracting situation in the Midwest, four competing hospitals had formed a marketing network. One of the hospitals had a strong reputation, was cost-effective, and was well received by contracting employers. The other three were not as attractive to employers. By taking a position that all four hospitals must have contracts or none would be available, the hospital with the strong reputation lost a potential opportunity because the employers refused to contract with the other three hospitals. Clearly, the hospital with the strong reputation would have benefited if it had the flexibility to contract independently.

Political Issues

Direct contracts between hospitals and employers can cause political controversies in some communities. Political issues are likely to arise in contracting situations when the purchaser is a coalition of employers that are fairly powerful within the marketplace. A hospital must analyze the political climate surrounding its relationship with the group of purchasers or the individual purchaser to determine how the political climate may affect the overall goals of the contract.

A primary issue in gauging the political climate of the contract is whether or not the purchaser group or individual employer is attempting to develop a cooperative relationship with long-term, positive goals or whether a quick fix is the objective. The reactions of the medical staff to the contracting process is also important.

The politics of contracting are affected by the relationships with hospital board members who may be a part of the employer group, the community's perception of this contracting process, and the issue of cost shifting to other employers or other private payers not involved in the contract. The situation is further complicated when the hospital itself is a member of a contracting coalition.

Members of the hospital board affiliated with employers seeking to contract may find themselves in a conflict-of-interest situation that could require their resignation from either the hospital board or the coalition. This situation has occurred in several communities in which employers are involved in direct contracts.

The community's perception and other employers' perceptions of cost shifting that may result from individual contracting may pose yet another political problem. If a hospital is contracting with one employer represented on its board and not another, the noncontracting employer may think that it is the object of increased cost shifting. Resolution of these types of problems varies by hospital and by community. In highly competitive markets, problems related to cost shifting may be insignificant.

Another political issue for hospitals contracting directly with employers has to do with the perceptions of competing hospitals and other organizations (PPOs and HMOs). Competitor relationships may be further complicated by the hospital's membership in a "competing" provider organization. This situation is occurring more frequently as hospitals continue to contract with multiple PPOs and HMOs. How the rates proposed to individual employers look in comparison with rates negotiated with PPOs or HMOs has a political impact on the hospital. In some cases, the individual hospitals have given an employer better terms because of the employer's ability to deliver a defined market. This situation can have a negative impact on the marketing abilities of PPOs in which the hospital is also a member.

The size of a community is relevant to the political intricacies of contracting with employers. Smaller communities may present more political problems for hospitals, which themselves are often the largest employers in town or otherwise have a firm feeling of community commitment.

Each community and each hospital has a unique political climate. Issues involving medical staff and board relations, community perception, and other hospital affiliations all have an impact on the direct contracting process.

Management Information Systems Requirements

The availability of data is always an important issue in direct employer contracting. To monitor contract performance, the employer or coalition needs utilization and cost information, and the hospital needs information on the financial and utilization impact related to contracts. A thorough review of the hospital's current internal management information system (MIS) is a first step in the process of determining if it can meet contract requirements for data. Among data-generating capabilities desired by purchasers are specific types of coding, including ICD-9, CPT-4, and in some cases, diagnosis-related groups (DRG). The ability to capture and sort information on an employer-specific, and not just payer-specific, basis is required as is the ability to generate reports on utilization and cost that are tailored to the purchaser's requirements.

When evaluating the hospital's current system, the cost of any needed refinements should figure into the financial feasibility of contracting. This cost may be arrived at through cost estimates for required systems modifications that can be provided by MIS staff or consultants.

Several resources are available to hospitals needing assistance in developing or refining data systems. They include consulting firms and software systems available for purchase. Also, hospitals should consider the option of developing a cooperative working relationship with purchasers to set up an MIS that would be useful to all parties involved.

Data from the MIS are used to support the contract monitoring process. The internal contract monitoring process for a hospital includes the assessment of hospital risk on a long-term, ongoing basis; financial performance of the contract; physician influence on cost; and an evaluation of utilization management programs, including preadmission certification, concurrent review, retrospective review, and case management. The ongoing purpose for contract monitoring is to determine the effectiveness of contracted arrangements. The analysis of financial data, utilization rates, and political issues (both medical and nonmedical) are important to this process. When the data analysis indicates that the contracted arrangements may create problems, the hospital may want to renegotiate certain contract terms or terminate the contract if the administrative costs, publicity, and market share do not warrant the level of financial commitment that may be required of it.

Various kinds of information are required for contract monitoring. The quantity of completed reviews must be monitored, and reports detailing the results of these reviews should be prepared. Hospital billing systems may need to be more automated, especially when an employer requires a paperless system. Figure 4-4 lists a standardized set of data elements that providers collect according to employer. Many contractors ask hospitals to provide some of these data elements through reports and through billing requirements (sample data reports for contract monitoring are discussed in chapter 1).

Quality Assurance and Utilization Management Systems

Comprehensive quality assurance and utilization management are important issues that enter into direct contracting with employers. Employers have two primary concerns and responsibilities when selecting and contracting with providers:

- Ensuring high-quality care for employees
- Managing the provision of services to ensure cost-effectiveness

Employers take seriously the responsibility for selecting providers. No benefits manager wants to offer employees medical services that

Figure 4-4. List of Health Care Data Elements Classified by Importance

General Health Care Data Elements

Essential

Patient's name

Patient's ZIP code

Patient's Social Security or identification number

Patient's date of birth

Patient's sex

Patient's relationship to insured

Insured's name

Insured's Social Security or identification number

Insured's sex

Insured's date of birth

Insured's identification number

Employer's name

Employer's location (ZIP code)

Medical facility's name

Place of service (for example, inpatient hospital, outpatient hospital, ambulatory care center, doctor's office)

Type of service (for example, medical, surgical, maternal, psychiatric, alcohol)

Medical facility's identification number (federal tax number)

Patient's claim number

Attending physician's or provider's name

Provider type (for example, physician, osteopath, podiatrist, optometrist, chiropractor, psychologist, physical therapist)

Attending physician's or provider's federal tax number

Date of admission or visit

Date of discharge

Principal diagnosis (5-digit ICD-9-CM)

(continued)

Figure 4-4.—continued

General Health Care Data Elements—continued

Essential—continued

Secondary diagnosis (5-digit ICD-9-CM)

Principal procedure (4-digit ICD-9-CM or 5-digit CPT-4)

Secondary procedure (4-digit ICD-9-CM or 5-digit CPT-4)

Date of principal procedure

Date of secondary procedure

Total room and board charges

Total ancillary charges

Facility's bill from date

Facility's bill to date

Type of facility's bill (interim or final)

Detail of attending physician's or other provider's procedures (CPT-4, dates, charges)

Type of attending physician's or other provider's bill (interim or final)

Desirable

Insured's classification (for example, hourly, salaried)

Insured's employment status (full-time, part-time, disabled, retiree)

Insured's job title

Type of medical facility (for example, hospital, skilled nursing facility, home health care)

Attending physician's or provider's specialty

Other physicians' or providers' names

Other physicians' or providers' type (for example, physician, osteopath, podiatrist, optometrist, chiropractor, psychologist, physical therapist)

Other physicians' or providers' identification numbers

Other physicians' or providers' specialties

Type of admission (for example, emergency, elective, newborn)

Admission status (for example, first admission, transfer from acute care facility, readmission)

(continued)

Figure 4-4.—continued

General Health Care Data Elements—continued

Desirable—continued

Date of admission to intensive care

Date of transfer from intensive care

Patient's discharge status or place of discharge (for example, alive, home self-care, skilled nursing facility, psychiatric facility, alcohol facility, deceased)

Additional secondary diagnoses (5-digit ICD-9-CM)

Additional secondary procedures (4-digit ICD-9-CM or 5-digit CPT-4)

Date of secondary procedures

Detail of routine charges (for example, intensive care, private, semiprivate)

Detail of ancillary charges (for example, pharmacy, radiology, pathology, operating room, medical supplies)

Ineligible and noncovered charges

Reasonable and customary reductions

Coordination-of-benefits dollars

Deductible

Coinsurance

Amount paid to medical facility

Detail of attending physician's and other providers' procedures (CPT-4, dates, amount paid)

Eligibility Data Elements

Essential

Insured's name

Insured's Social Security number

Insured's date of birth

Insured's sex

Insured's employment date

Insured's termination date

(continued)

Figure 4-4.—continued

Eligibility Data Elements—continued

Essential—continued

Insured's coverage effective date

Insured's coverage termination date

Spouse's Social Security number

Spouse's date of birth

Spouse's sex

Spouse's coverage effective date

Spouse's coverage termination date

Other dependents' date of birth

Other dependents' sex

Other dependents' coverage effective date

Other dependents' coverage termination date

Employer's name

Employer's location (division or ZIP code)

Insured's classification (for example, hourly, salaried)

Insured's employment status (full-time, part-time, disabled, retiree)

Desirable

Job title or occupation

Other insurance coverage

Other insurance plan sponsor (for example, Blue Cross-Blue Shield, commercial carrier, Medicare)

Other insurance plan benefit contact (for example, spouse, parent)

Other insurance plan effective date

Other insurance plan termination date

are perceived as being of less than optimum quality. In addition, employers must also take into consideration the potential for legal liability that stems from providing employees with incentives to seek care from specific providers. This liability may further encourage employers to be selective in contracting. Accountability, appropriateness of care provided, and cost of care remain overall employer concerns.

Employers do not generally wish to be in the role of determining quality. Rather they wish to ensure that providers are effectively monitoring their own provisions of medical services. Although many employers now realize the key importance of quality to cost-effectiveness, they are not in a position to evaluate it. They wish to simply monitor quality review by providers.

In addition to managing quality, managing service utilization is important in employer contracting. Employers may seek to ensure appropriate utilization through third-party reviewers or through delegated review.

From the hospital's perspective, the pros and cons of delegated versus nondelegated review should be considered in each contract. *Delegated review* is performed by the hospital. If the contract calls for a delegated review, the hospital should get satisfactory answers to the following questions:

- Does the hospital have a data system in place to fulfill requirements, or must data functions be completed manually?
- Can current hospital staff fulfill contract requirements for utilization management staffing and operations?
- What are the administrative costs of performing the contracted utilization management functions?
- Are alterations in current preadmission certification, concurrent review, or case management criteria required?
- How closely will employers monitor the hospital's review process?
- How does physician compliance with the hospital's utilization management program affect the contract?
- Can the hospital charge a fee for the service?

Nondelegated review is a review by an outside third-party organization or employer. If the contract calls for nondelegated review, the hospital must get satisfactory answers to the following questions:

- Who makes preadmission certification and length-of-stay decisions, and how credible are the criteria when compared with other standardized criteria?
- Are physicians and hospitals bound to decisions of the reviewing organization in terms of absolute payment determination?
- How does the appeals process function for physicians and for the hospital, and what are the payment implications?
- How do the imposed criteria relate to the hospital's own criteria and standards for admission and length of stay?
- What administrative duties are required of the hospital, and what is the overall cost?
- What types of information will the hospital receive from the reviewing group?
- What are the disciplinary actions related to noncompliance?

Utilization management and quality assurance are important negotiation issues for employers. A hospital is well prepared if it develops internal systems that can facilitate delegated review. Generally, a hospital, in conjunction with its medical staff, prefers to be in charge of monitoring the way care is managed in its facility. However, in some cases, nondelegated review may be preferred, especially when the hospital, for political reasons, does not wish to dictate to its medical staff; when the cost of review functions is high; or when the hospital wishes to gain credibility by having an outside review performed.

Operational Issues

Operational issues in direct contracting are generally related to billing procedures, data requirements, utilization management process, employee communication, and any committee responsibilities or other requirements of an employer. All responsibilities should be clearly delineated in the contract.

Often overlooked are the following important contracting issues related to operations:

- Which party bears responsibility for verification of covered benefits?

- How does the employee identification process operate?
- How does the hospital bill for copayments and deductibles?
- How does the hospital bill for the services of hospital-based physicians?
- How is payment for on-call physicians handled?
- Who is responsible for delivering marketing materials to employees?
- Who is responsible for the development and distribution of a provider directory?
- How are payment schedules administered, and who calculates payment?
- What is the dispute resolution process?
- How do requirements for coordination and maintenance of benefits differ from the hospital's normal procedures?
- How is patient confidentiality covered in the contract?

Other operational issues for hospitals contracting directly with employers are ongoing management systems operation, contract monitoring, utilization management operation, interface with claims administrators, and coordination and integration with physician organizations and other services and networks.

Negotiations

Each negotiation process and contract is unique. This point cannot be stressed enough. Achieving the goal of a mutually satisfactory relationship can be a satisfying process in direct contracting; sometimes, such a relationship can be more achievable when contracting directly with an employer than when working through a PPO, HMO, or insurance carrier. Employers may be more inclined to develop cooperative arrangements through negotiations. Often, insurers or other groups simply offer a contract on a take-it-or-leave-it basis. Omitting the middle party allows for direct discussions between purchaser and supplier.

A negotiation process that can prove beneficial to both providers and employers is displayed in figure 4-5 and discussed in the following sections. Some arrangements may, in the course of negotiations, be determined to be too administratively cumbersome or too costly to pursue, or they may result in competitive disadvantage for the hospital. Hospitals

Figure 4-5. Overview of Hospital Negotiation and Contracting Process

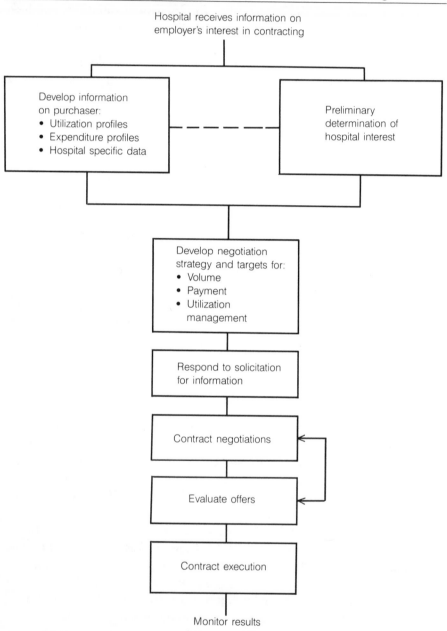

should evaluate the potential of a contract from the onset of negotiations and continue to reevaluate issues as negotiations progress.

Preparation for Negotiations

The hospital's preparations for the negotiation process are generally in response to a specific employer request but may be initiated as an ongoing strategic marketing activity of the hospital. This preparation involves several steps:

- Developing pertinent information about potential purchasers
- Developing negotiation targets and priorities
- Responding to solicitation for information
- Forming a negotiating team
- Determining issues that require termination of negotiations and contracting

Development of Purchaser Information

Gathering detailed information on an employer or group is vital to successful negotiation strategies. Information on the purchaser's goals and objectives, cost concerns, benefits design, employee age and sex demographics, geographic dispersion of employees, administrative capabilities, timetables, and clout may be collected from several sources. These sources include the hospital's own data base, the local chamber of commerce, association and coalition directories, and the employers themselves.

Following the completion of the initial research and perhaps a brief initial meeting with the prospective purchaser, the hospital should try to answer these questions:

- How important is this contract to the hospital in relation to the following?
  - Current volume
  - Potential volume
  - Political issues
  - Perception of other purchasers
- How much potential market gain or retention can the hospital expect?
- Can the hospital price at a level that is acceptable to this purchaser and still achieve profit goals?

- Is risk sharing appropriate with this employer?
- What types of payment arrangements can the purchaser administer?
- How much information does the purchaser have on this hospital?
- Is the purchaser looking for a long-term relationship or a "quick fix"?

Negotiation Targets

Prior to actual negotiation sessions, the hospital should set appropriate primary, secondary, and tertiary negotiation targets based on its information on the potential purchaser. Examples of such targets are:

- Guaranteed volume (primary)
  Variable prices based on volume (secondary)
  Ability to retain patients at a fair price (tertiary)
- Delegated UR, hospital controlled (primary)
  Partially delegated UR (secondary)
  Acceptable criteria and process, outside UR firm (tertiary)

Additional priorities and targets should be established for pricing, incentive design, and competitor involvement. Trade-offs based on equitable arrangements can be negotiated. However, any trade-offs should be based on the goal of developing a mutually satisfactory relationship.

Solicitation for Information

Employers frequently send out requests for proposals from providers. If the hospital is interested in contracting, its responses should be:

- Concise and complete, furnishing all requested information in the specified format
- Prepared so that the request for proposal can be used as a marketing tool as well as an information source

Negotiating Team

Appropriate team members and team style are important in negotiations. Most employers and hospitals are familiar with union and vendor negotiations and are attuned to fairly sophisticated negotiation processes. Employers may use similar strategies in hospital negotiations.

The composition of the hospital's negotiating team depends on the purchaser's importance. At a minimum, staff with complete knowledge of hospital attributes, a finance representative, and a UR specialist should be on the team. The employer assesses the hospital's level of interest by the structure and responsiveness of negotiation participants. If phone calls are not returned and meetings are cancelled or attended by low-ranking staff members, a negative signal is sent to the employer.

Termination of Negotiations

Prior to the beginning of negotiations, the hospital should determine the issues that may require the termination of negotiations. These issues should be listed in order of priority as they relate to targeted goals, and the team must be prepared to individually evaluate each issue as the need arises.

The following are some issues that may require the termination of negotiations:

- Excessive administration burdens
- Excessive financial risk
- Rates well below acceptable targeted range
- Most favored nation clause
- Lack of volume potential
- Exclusivity requirements
- Indemnification
- Demands for additional medical staff
- Patient confidentiality issues

Negotiating Tips

The following negotiating tips may help a hospital involved in direct employer contracting:

- Know the current volume of business this employer represents for the institution before negotiations begin. Revenues from employers that range from 2 to 5 percent put the employer in a strong negotiating position.

- Be responsive to requests for information. If the information requested is inappropriate, provide substitute information.
- Be frank and open about the hospital's attributes and constraints. For example, if the hospital provides much uncompensated care, talk about it and have data to substantiate the claim.
- Do not do a "glitz" marketing job. Employers are seeking knowledge and sincerity, not slick marketers.
- Ask for demographic and other information and emphasize its importance in arriving at risk-sharing arrangements.
- Be flexible in contracting.
- Be ready to do some educating. Employers may need assistance in understanding some delivery-of-care issues. Their understanding can be extremely useful to the hospital.

Conclusion

Direct contracting with employers or groups of employers is an important new concept in the purchasing and selling of health care services. As health care becomes an increasingly market-driven industry, these contracting activities will be more prevalent.

Direct employer contracting represents a new and sometimes advantageous way for hospitals to access private-payer markets. It requires careful planning and negotiations as well as a thorough evaluation of the hospital's strengths and weaknesses.

Direct employer contracting may negate the need for developing or depending on PPO and HMO contracts to retain or expand market share. It provides one method for directly accessing the purchasers of health care services. The following are key hospital considerations in direct employer contracting:

- The true advantages or disadvantages of each employer contract should be carefully evaluated, and the long-term as well as the short-term impact of the contract should be carefully considered.
- Ongoing monitoring of the contract and communication with the employer is crucial to the success of the arrangement.
- The ability to work directly with employers, and directly with their employees, can provide significant marketing advantages to the hospital.

Chapter 5

Implementing PPO Contracts

Introduction

A strategic environmental analysis, as described in part I, should indicate overall strategies for the hospital to consider. Hospitals must carefully evaluate all options available and determine the most appropriate and beneficial approaches to follow. This chapter concentrates on preferred provider organizations (PPOs), which can be broadly defined as organizations that facilitate arrangements between health care providers and group purchasers of health care services to ensure the delivery of cost-effective, high-quality health care services.

Many hospitals have embarked on strategies to contract with all PPOs in the marketplace to avoid being excluded from any market segment. Others, wary of administrative costs and reputation implications, have been more selective.

Hospitals must develop a detailed evaluation criteria list with which to judge all PPO contract offerings. This chapter suggests pertinent evaluation criteria and reviews several specific considerations that providers must resolve if they are to contract effectively with a PPO. Much of the discussion of chapter 4, on direct employer contracts, is also applicable to the PPO contracting process.

Contracting Team

Contracting with PPOs requires a hospital management team that is dedicated to overseeing and facilitating planning and monitoring processes similar to those recommended in chapter 4 for direct employer contracting. Briefly, the contracting team described in chapter 4 includes the contract manager, chief financial officer (CFO), marketing director, attorney, utilization review (UR) manager, and hospital chief executive officer (CEO). In addition, the data systems manager is an ad hoc member of the team.

The operation of a PPO is similar and in many respects identical to that of an insurance company. The day-to-day management tasks require personnel who have experience in insurance management: sales, underwriting, enrollment, benefits design, and customer relations. Therefore, hospitals contracting with existing PPOs or with PPOs under development must understand the insurance industry if they are to effectively negotiate arrangements that are beneficial to the hospital.

When selecting or reviewing PPO programs for possible contracting, a hospital should evaluate the structure and staffing of the PPO. Managing a PPO is a major undertaking that demands full-time commitment from its managers. The hospital should make sure that the PPO has an adequate staff to cover various support functions. Administrative personnel are needed to handle accounting and payroll tasks, employee benefits, materials supply, and so forth. After the PPO is incorporated, legal staff are required for reviewing the printed marketing materials, drafting contracts with employers, and reviewing individual contracts. Another specialist required is a benefits consultant to help the PPO staff determine how the program can be integrated with various benefits plans required by employers. Actuarial consultants are needed to prepare the premium-rate quotation that most employers require before they can evaluate the competitiveness of the PPO's product offering. These quotations, which are based on employee demographic information, help the PPO and the hospital evaluate various pricing arrangements that may be offered to determine the financial risk to be assumed by each party to the contract. Finally, advertising and public relations personnel are required to create a coordinated program theme and to develop an effective marketing program.

Marketing Issues

Among the purposes of a hospital's strategic marketing plan should be the facilitation of long-term relationships with selected purchasers. One way such relationships can be accomplished is through PPO contracting. To develop a strategy for approaching various market segments, the hospital must first find out who its present patients are, where they work, what kinds of services they use, how profitable they are to the hospital, and the level of severity of their illnesses. This information is then compared with the marketing plan of an area PPO to determine if the hospital's affiliation with that PPO meets the hospital's objective of solidifying long-term purchaser relationships or if the PPO's marketing plan encourages current patients to use other hospitals or facilities, thereby eroding the hospital's present patient base. This process is a key factor in the selection of PPOs for potential contracting opportunities.

A hospital must develop a marketing plan that retains present business and outlines a strategy for attracting profitable new patients who represent the minimum possible financial risk. Historically, hospitals have classified patients according to whether payment was made by Medicare, Medicaid, Blue Cross, commercial insurance, or other payers. Now hospitals must identify patients by employer and analyze the market share that each employer can bring to the hospital. The process of identifying patients by employer leads to the segmentation of the market by the type of vehicle used by the employer to provide its health care benefits, such as self-insurance, commercial insurance, or health maintenance organizations (HMOs). A unique marketing strategy is required for each of these market segments.

The hospital's marketing staff must clearly understand what services are available from the PPO and how these services may be better used by prospective purchasers. To do this, the hospital's marketing staff should know as much about prospective PPO clients as possible. The marketing staff must have knowledge of benefits plans and their limitations, geographic dispersion of an employers' employees, locations of various plants and offices, and the employers' current cost of health care services. The gathering of this information is discussed in detail in chapter 4.

Hospitals will find that a PPO can supplement and support the planning, marketing, and community relations functions of the hospital, and the hospital can do the same for the PPO. A PPO can be an ideal marketing vehicle for a hospital and can be integrated with other related marketing functions to meet the hospital's overall goals and objectives.

Financial Planning Issues

Hospitals should be aware of how the PPO is being capitalized. Capitalization may determine the marketing strategy of the PPO and the ability of the plan to attract new members who will use the participating hospitals' services. Additional financial planning issues relate to the negotiated payment levels and risk levels. Internal administrative costs and overall financial impact of the loss or gain of patients under the terms of the contract are discussed in previous chapters. Each of these issues must be individually evaluated for each PPO contract negotiated.

Capitalization Expense

The developmental costs and ongoing administrative costs of a PPO are often financed by member hospitals. How a contracting PPO is sponsored and financed determines the hospital's share of administrative costs. In recent years, many hospitals have created corporate entities that permit financial flexibility in contracting with PPOs and provide for the development of other competitive plans.

The capitalization of the PPO may require contracting hospitals to participate in financing developmental costs of the PPO through either a one-time or an ongoing fee assessment. Ongoing administrative costs of a PPO are frequently funded by preferred provider membership fees, both initial and annual; by continued financial support from the parent corporation; or by payment for allied services that the PPO may offer, such as the services of a claims administrator. Many hospitals consider such PPO fees as marketing expenses for the hospital.

Many PPOs believe that employers will pay a monthly administrative PPO fee. A PPO that is developed and marketed by an insurance carrier may build these fees into its premiums. However, such an arrangement is difficult to market directly to employers unless significant additional direct services are provided by the PPO to the employer. Employers will pay for services that are necessary for the administration of their benefits plans but may not simply pay for the privilege of using a PPO service that is ill-defined or not relevant to the employer.

Payment Issues and Assumption of Risk

A primary issue that faces all hospitals contracting with PPOs or other organizations is payment for services and the relationship of various pricing alternatives to the amount of risk assumed by the providers or the PPO. Even though many PPOs have stated that they do not assume risk, their contracting hospitals accept some form of per case, per diem, or diagnosis rate as payment in full. Participating hospital and physician providers must thoroughly understand the level of risk associated with these payment arrangements and develop corporate policies to guide the hospital's marketing staff in negotiations with PPOs and other purchasers.

Many forms of creative payment arrangements fall somewhere between full charges (no risk) and capitation rates (total risk) for both hospitals and physicians. The method that is best for both hospital and PPO must take into account the PPO's capability to assume financial risk, the marketability of the approach, and the PPO's or the insurance company partner's capability of underwriting the risk. Hospitals must carefully evaluate each offered contract in terms of associated risk. Experience data should be provided by the PPO to the hospital to assist in this evaluation.

The amount of risk sharing varies significantly among purchasers with the same payment arrangement because of the different age and sex composition of the covered populations; the purchaser's subscriber penetration, benefits plan design, and effectiveness of employee incentives; and utilization rate of the covered population. A PPO that properly understands these issues knows that it needs actuarial assessment of the risk for every major client with whom it negotiates some payment rate other than full charges or percentage discount. This assessment is necessary to shield both their contracting hospitals and the PPO from inappropriate risk levels.

Organizational Structure

A PPO may be an independent, freestanding corporation organized either for profit or not for profit or as a subsidiary of a parent corporation. Hospital integration into the arrangement can be as a shareholder, subsidiary, parent, or contractor.

The organizational structure of a PPO can take many forms of varying complexity, but all of these forms are influenced by two factors: motivation of the sponsoring entity itself and the entity's ability to share financial risk. Currently existing models are based on sponsorship or control by different legal entities through joint ventures, partnerships, or other legal arrangements.

The organizational structures of a PPO generally fall within three categories: simple, fully integrated, and shared health options purchasing (SHOP) plan. Figures 5-1, 5-2, and 5-3 illustrate these structures in detail. Figure 5-1 shows a simple PPO structure in which a separate legal entity is formed by a sponsoring group that has for-profit or not-for-profit status. This entity operates as a broker, contracting with selected providers for medical services and with employers or insurance

Figure 5-1. Simple PPO

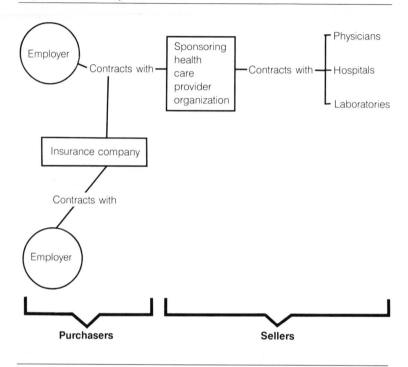

Figure 5-2. Horizontally and Vertically Integrated PPO

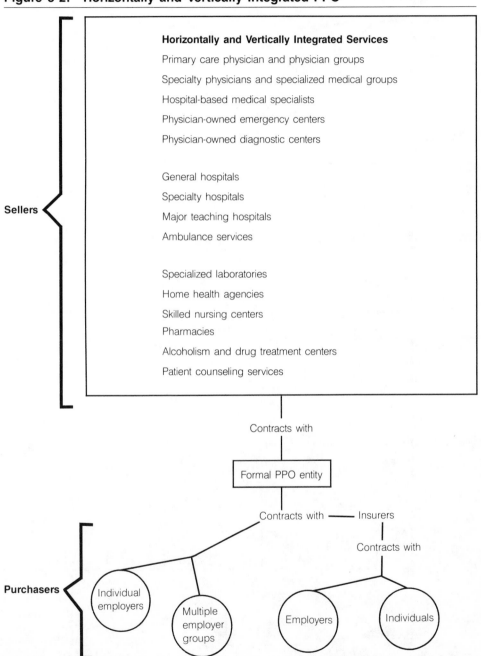

Figure 5-3.   SHOP Plan

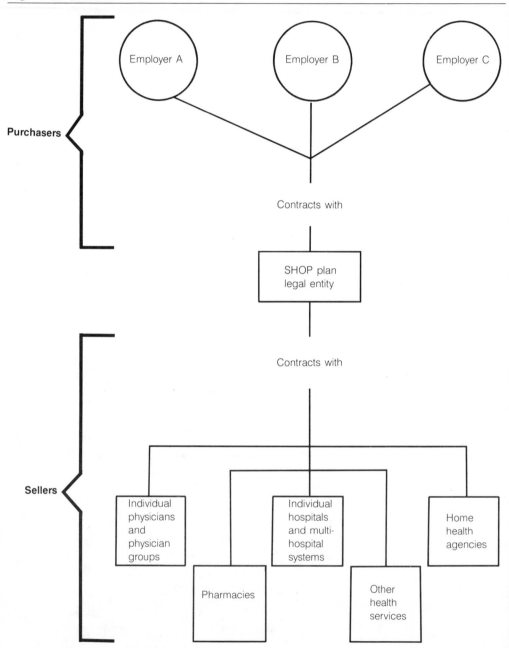

companies to sell those services. Figure 5-2, which is a horizontally and vertically integrated model, is organized by a network of providers under contract or as equity owners of the PPO. The PPO again contracts with purchasers for the provision of services. This structure is often more marketable because of the vertical integration of services. The shared health options purchasing (SHOP) plan structure shown in figure 5-3 is described in chapter 4. This model is sponsored and controlled by the purchasing group.

The organizational design of the PPO is often influenced by the ability or willingness of the contracting parties to share economic risk. In addition, the appropriate structure of the PPO is influenced by legal restraints, the political environment, and the desired control and flexibility of the hospital.

Political Issues

The decision to contract with a PPO must be carefully weighed against the realities of the political issues affecting the success or failure of such arrangements. The immediate community served by the hospital should be given first consideration. The issues of competition and health care cost containment as perceived by purchasers of services should be properly evaluated. Hospitals must evaluate the political implications of their market assessment studies and their physicians' concerns within the context of purchasers' requirements.

The hospital must consider the initiatives of all other medical providers within its market area and evaluate the impact of any competing programs. It must consider current support relationships and affiliations with other medical providers and evaluate potential responses to the PPO program.

The involvement of physicians in decision making is always necessary and is especially important in politically charged PPO contracting situations. Contracts with PPOs often impose constraints on physicians, such as utilization review requirements, referral restrictions, and payment limits.

Management Information Systems Requirements

Every PPO and employer has its own benefits plan requirements and different levels of incentives for employees to use preferred providers.

A hospital's information system must be able to implement and monitor all variations of benefits requirements in preferred provider arrangements in order to administer the contract requirements and respond to contract renewals or modifications.

The hospital's data systems must be comprehensive and must have the capability of profiling costs and utilization patterns to complement the management information requirements of the PPO. A hospital must be able to collect data by employer benefit plans; number of admissions; emergency department visits; outpatient services received; ambulatory surgical patients; and utilization of special services such as psychiatry, rehabilitation, skilled nursing, home care, or hospice. A hospital must also be able to break down its total service load according to PPO contract and then employer and determine which services are being purchased most often so that it can evaluate the PPO's marketing program and develop its own marketing program to strengthen current service volume and increase participation in programs selected for promotion. A comprehensive system is also required when the financial arrangement between hospital and PPO involves any form of financial risk sharing.

Utilization management information collected by the hospital that is specific to physician practice patterns assists the PPO in selecting physicians who practice cost-efficient and cost-effective medicine. The practice patterns of these physicians in turn contribute to a positive image of the hospital's overall performance. In turn, contracting PPOs should be providing hospitals with data on practice patterns, market share, and utilization of services.

Many sophisticated employers require PPOs to have effective UR and peer review programs and submit reports directly to them on their employees' experiences. These employers are interested in monitoring their employees' use of health care services and the respective costs of these services.

Integration with Payer Systems

Hospitals contracting with a PPO should evaluate whether the PPO fully understands the employer's claims administration system constraints and has created a program that is flexible enough to produce the desired results. Many PPOs develop elaborate program features, including benefits and financial risk arrangements, only to find that the systems cannot be administered by employers' claims administrators. Most claims processing systems lack the design flexibility to process creative preferred provider arrangements. Prior to contracting with a PPO, the hospital can request information regarding claims processing methodology and ask its own claims administrator if it would be able to handle the payments under the proposed arrangements.

Some PPOs have chosen to create a claims processing system that is as flexible as the marketplace requires and that provides necessary management information to both hospitals and employers. A problem with this approach is that the employer's current claims administrator may be unwilling to cooperate with this PPO or may charge an additional administrative fee for processing claims. As a result, the employer may not contract with the PPO.

Furthermore, creating a PPO that has this processing capability can be extremely resource intensive. Hospitals that are asked to participate should be wary. Even though this type of PPO may have a market advantage, it can be costly to the hospital that is asked to contribute to the PPO's administrative expenses.

A PPO should capture information on the administrative capabilities of major insurance carriers, claims administrator, and self-administered claims systems within their service area. A PPO must consider what limitations or flexibility exist in the marketplace and what type of PPO system is marketable to employers. Hospitals should examine the PPOs capability in this area carefully because such capability could be a key factor in the marketability of the PPOs.

Quality Assurance and Utilization Management Systems

Many sophisticated purchasers place more emphasis on quality of health care and effective utilization management than on negotiated price reductions. However, many employers weigh price and quality equally, and some consider price alone. Therefore, hospitals must have quality assurance and utilization management programs whose effectiveness can be demonstrated to contractors that use these systems as selection criteria for provider panel development.

To be effective, these programs must provide for the exchange of utilization and quality information among all parties: hospitals and physicians, hospitals and PPOs, physicians and PPOs, and PPOs and purchasers. This free exchange permits all participants to monitor the effectiveness of the program.

Many PPOs permit employers to participate in peer review committees by being present at meetings when their employees' cases are being reviewed. Employers are often appreciative of the opportunity to participate in the utilization management process and may reciprocate by supplying hospitals with other utilization and cost data.

Hospitals have various methods for demonstrating the soundness of their utilization management program to contracting PPOs. Many contracting hospitals have furnished their latest Joint Commission on Accreditation of Hospitals report to PPOs and employers that have requested information relating to quality assurance. Other hospitals have reviewed their quality assurance committee procedures and results with PPOs and employers. As hospitals expand medical services into alternative delivery modes, they must also plan for effective quality assurance and utilization management programs that monitor and report all patient care activity.

Operational Issues

When a hospital signs a PPO contract, operational issues that the PPO and hospital should discuss include data requirements, frequency of reporting the data, and structure or format for reporting. Other pertinent matters are utilization management procedures and requirements, payment time frames, admissions procedures, and methodologies for hospital contract monitoring and renegotiation. Admissions procedures, including types of identification, level of benefits, and any other procedures required of a patient (such as second-opinion surgery programs), should be fully spelled out in a hospital operating procedures manual.

A hospital should examine six key areas as they relate to PPO operations: management, legal, provider relations, finances, marketing, and administrative services. After a contract is signed, these areas need to be carefully monitored on an ongoing basis.

Management issues, which revolve around the development and implementation by the PPO of policies and procedures covering all operations, should be carefully studied for their effect on the hospital. Added to policy issues is the implementation of an effective management information system and reporting structure. Utilization review programs and controls to examine include patient monitoring and tracking capabilities.

Hospitals should evaluate PPO operations to determine their legality and any potential liability that may relate back to the hospital. The legal staff should be reviewing on an ongoing basis all court decisions and new regulations, both state and federal, as they apply to the PPO. Marketing materials should also be reviewed to prevent misrepresentation and minimize any potential antitrust problems.

Ongoing provider relations requires contracting hospitals and physicians to participate in continuing educational and training sessions for office staff and new physicians as they enter the program. Program updates, enrollment figures, status of marketing efforts, and other pertinent information needs to be furnished to the providers regularly.

Financial considerations include PPO interface and coordination with all of the different administrators representing employers participating in the PPO. Every administrator has different administrative arrangements and interface requirements. Any problems need to be mutually resolved to the benefit of the PPO and the employer and communicated to the preferred providers. In addition, the hospital should review the internal financial statements of the PPO and ensure that the PPO is monitoring the ongoing level of financial risk assumed by the provider payment mechanism.

Marketing issues for the PPO involve the design and implementation of programs aimed at developing a defined market and creating favorable community awareness and support, including public relations functions. Other important marketing issues are the integration of ancillary medical services into the PPO product furnished outside the provider setting and the establishment of effective networks that are attractive to the employers. The PPO's marketing staff, either in conjunction with hospital staff or separately, is also responsible for the ongoing employer staff training on the PPO program. Hospitals participating in the PPO should evaluate the PPO's marketing capability both initially and on an ongoing basis.

In the early stages of development, the PPO may have to use contracted help or consultants to assist in management until it can justify adding full-time management staff. The management and organizers of a PPO must be realistic about expected marketing results and must carefully target prospective purchasers. Long-term projections may be more acceptable to the developers or sponsors of the PPO than short-term results. Hospitals actively participating in a PPO should ask the PPO for their short-term and long-term marketing plan and evaluate if these goals are realistic.

The evaluation of administrative services offered to contracting hospitals is also important. If the PPO offers billing, benefits verification, education, or other services, the price of those services should be evaluated against their value to the hospital.

Negotiations

As PPO contracting increases and PPO membership continues to grow, hospitals need to develop an overall strategy for contracting based on the competitiveness of the marketplace. The philosophy underlying the basic strategy may be one of several: contracting with all PPOs, contracting with a selected few based on definite criteria for selection, or not contracting with PPOs. The appropriate strategy depends on the demographics of the marketplace and the strategic plan a hospital has for maintaining competitiveness.

As hospitals are inundated with multiple PPO and other contracts, they must develop specific criteria and evaluation processes to select those PPOs that will have a positive impact on the hospital. These criteria should evaluate the PPO organization itself and the contract terms.

Knowledge of PPO Organization

Prior to negotiations, the hospital should evaluate the PPO organization itself. This evaluation of the PPO should include:

- Organizational structure, management structure, governance structure, and tax status
- Short-term and long-term financial stability
- Quality issues within the PPO, both historically and currently
- Utilization management program and its effect on accessibility to care for members

- Information systems and ability to share or desire to share information it gathers with the hospital
- Ability to deliver a new market share to the hospital or retain current market share, including evaluation of other hospitals under contract and their competitiveness with the hospital considering a contract as well as the PPO's overall market share in the community
- Examination of any political reasons to contract or not to contract with a PPO, including religious mission or philosophy or other special issues

Figure 5-4 lists additional evaluation criteria.

Evaluation of Contract Provisions

In addition to overall payment provisions, the PPO contract should be evaluated in terms of specific issues, such as use of a hospital's name in marketing, contract termination provision applying to both parties, any volume guarantees or rate arrangements that are tied to a volume percentage, and UR requirements. Other issues of importance are the level of services being contracted for (specialty only, full-service, or extended vertically integrated services); the role of physicians or physician organization; the responsibility for verification of benefits; and administrative procedures such as billing, admissions, payment time frames, and the appropriate sources for distribution of information. Further, confidentiality of patient data should also be covered in a contract.

Traditionally, PPOs have contracted with hospitals on a discount-off-charges basis. Many PPOs are now moving to risk-sharing arrangements. A hospital must evaluate the short-term and long-term effects of these different payment arrangements on its internal cash flow. The positive or negative effects are based on the level of the hospital's risk and its ability to make a profit on that group of patients. Again, profitability is related to the age, sex, and geographic dispersion of the PPO client population. Also, at the end of each contract year, a hospital should consider an actuarial evaluation of its overall level of risk based on multiple risk-sharing contracts.

Negotiating Tips

Objectives for the hospital in the negotiation process should pertain to payment level and volume potential and maintenance of a level

Figure 5-4. Evaluation of a PPO (Success Factors)

- Thorough analysis of the marketplace
  - —Have they done it?
  - —What factors did they evaluate?
  - —How does the analysis relate to the hospital's analysis?
- Selection of reputable, cost-effective providers
  - —Hospital's competitors
  - —Hospitals with cost or reputation problems
- Effective utilization management program
  - —Elements: for example, preadmission certification, concurrent review, second-surgical opinion, discharge planning
  - —Ramifications for hospital
- Involvement of purchasers and providers in the development, a cooperative approach
  - —Advisory approach
  - —Purchasers in board positions
- Appropriate incentives for providers
  - —Fee schedules
  - —Bonus pools
  - —Shareholder status
  - —Other
- Incentives for consumers
  - —Plan design
  - —Risk sharing
  - —Incentives
- Appropriate geographic coverage: Providers in key market areas
- Financial stability
- Track record
  - —Utilization management
  - —Contracting
  - —Subscription
- Administrative staff expertise

of autonomy. The PPO negotiation process may be similar to that outlined in chapter 4 for direct employer contracting. However, key negotiation issues are:

- Assessing the PPO's importance and market power as related to the hospital
- Basing strategies for negotiation on the relative value of the PPO to the hospital
- Assessing administrative membership fees and determining the appropriateness of fees in relation to the services received
- Evaluating offered market-area exclusivity
- Creating arrangements that are positive for both the hospital and the PPO

Conclusion

Preferred provider programs present a challenge to hospitals that want to market their services to employers. Today's employers are becoming involved and informed purchasers of health care and are in a position to control their programs, which have been delegated to other parties in the past. With this changing involvement, PPOs are challenged to be as responsive and creative as their targeted employer clients. Therefore, product and service delivery capabilities and financial arrangements must be well designed, competitive, and responsive to employers' needs. If not, the PPO will lose out in the free competitive market. The following are key hospital considerations in PPO contracting:

- A knowledgeable, skilled management staff is important to the success of a hospital contracting with a PPO. A significant time commitment is required.
- Strategic market planning and product definition are crucial for the PPO and contracting hospitals.
- Financial planning and monitoring must continue on an ongoing basis. The hospital must determine the appropriateness of the contract and the financial stability of the PPO.
- Political problems, including community response and medical staff disputes, could arise from a hospital's involvement with PPOs.
- Risk sharing must be based on information; informed decision-making is the only appropriate option. The analysis of level of risk is an ongoing process.

Chapter 6

Implementing HMO and CMP Contracts

Introduction

In many marketplaces and communities, contracting with health main-tenance organizations (HMOs) has become a key element in the sur-vival of hospitals. As with preferred provider organizations (PPOs) and direct employer contracting, the level of the hospital's involvement in and commitment to various HMO initiatives depends on its overall stra-tegic marketing plan. In communities where HMO penetration is at the national average or higher, most hospitals choose to be involved in many HMO contracts. Hospitals that have considered developing their own HMOs have often learned that doing so is a time-consuming, expen-sive, and risky venture. Consequently, many hospitals prefer to contract with HMOs rather than starting their own HMO. This chapter discusses hospital contracting with HMOs and, like the preceding chapter, builds on many of the concepts and issues discussed in chapter 4.

An HMO is legally defined as a prepaid comprehensive medical plan that offers prescribed services to an enrolled population. Feder-ally qualified HMOs are eligible to contract with the Health Care Financing Administration (HCFA) to provide services to Medicare bene-ficiaries. Similarly, a competitive medical plan (CMP) offers prescribed services to an enrolled population for a prepaid fee. Federal certifica-tion entitles the CMP to contract with HCFA to provide services to Medicare beneficiaries without meeting the stricter guidelines applicable to federal qualification. However, CMPs are not granted some of the other benefits associated with federal qualification.

Congress developed the concept of CMPs to encourage compe-tition in health care delivery. The CMP program expands the num-ber of organizations that are eligible to provide prepaid health care to Medicare beneficiaries. Both CMPs and HMOs offer a mecha-nism to ensure that beneficiaries receive continuity of care and con-tinuity in the quality of care, and they give health care providers incentives to control costs. In general, the issues that are applicable to HMO contracting are also applicable to CMP contracting.

In determining the extent to which the hospital plans to become involved in HMO contracting, the hospital must always keep in mind that an HMO's primary goal is to control utilization of inpatient hospital services. A hospital's goal is often to increase or retain utilization of inpatient services. Therefore, when evaluating an HMO contract, a hospital needs to be able to forecast the HMO's ability to maintain or deliver a net increase in patient days. Hospitals must also take into consideration other service utilization by HMO members (for example, emergency, outpatient, and ancillary services) and the percentage of primary admitting physicians on staff who are contracting to provide services to HMO enrollees. A shift in their admitting patterns can significantly affect the hospital's overall utilization.

Contracting Team

One assigned staff member or a contracting team, as described in chapter 4, should be responsible for planning and following through with all of the contracting issues to be discussed in this chapter. All of the hospital staff involved in the process should have the necessary and appropriate skills and knowledge. The contract team, like the team described in chapters 4 and 5 (on contracting directly with employers and with PPOs respectively), may include the contract manager, chief financial officer, marketing director, utilization review (UR) manager, and chief executive officer. As mentioned in connection with these previous circumstances, the level of involvement of each is dependent on the negotiation approach of the HMO.

In contracting with HMOs, hospitals are sometimes placed in the reactive position of responding to a request for proposal or even to a less formal solicitation for information and price estimate. Hospital contracting teams must be prepared to respond to requests for proposals in a timely fashion.

Careful evaluation of financial and risk aspects of the contract, as well as the administrative responsibilities and utilization management approaches previously outlined in chapters 4 and 5, are key responsibilities of the team that negotiates and monitors HMO contracts. The contracting team must also monitor the quality of care delivered by the HMO and assess its reputation in the community. To be effective in its evaluation, the contracting team should understand the state and federal laws that apply to HMOs and CMPs.

Marketing Issues

When considering a contract with an HMO or CMP, a hospital should carefully evaluate the percentage of current patient days attributable to enrollees of the HMO or CMP, including Medicare beneficiaries, and forecast the hospital's ability to retain that patient-day level should it choose not to contract. A similar exercise should be completed for each HMO with which the hospital is currently contracting. The information needed to complete this task is derived from a market analysis as described in part I of this book and emphasized in chapter 4.

The hospital should beware of contracting a large percentage of patient days to only one or two HMOs. If the HMO represents a major portion of the hospital's total patient days, the financial power that it could exert over the hospital may be considerable.

Hospitals developing specific marketing plans for HMO contracting should, in addition to offering comprehensive services, look at specific hospital services or unbundled programs in such areas as substance abuse, wellness, outpatient services, specialty services, and ambulatory surgery to determine which products are of interest to HMOs and how best to market them. If the hospital is solicited to provide specialty care only, the potential risk to the hospital and the market volume the hospital can expect should be carefully estimated through an analysis of service costs as related to competitive market price. Throughout the planning process, the hospital should pinpoint its strengths and capitalize on their marketability. Careful market analysis identifies areas for competitive concentration.

Hospital staff involved in contracting should also evaluate the network of providers associated with an HMO and determine whether or not the hospital wants its name associated with the other partners or with the HMO organization itself. Part of such a determination involves looking at the financial stability and management expertise of the HMO.

Financial Planning Issues

Contracting with an HMO can be financially beneficial to a hospital when the HMO's marketing plan is consistent with the hospital's strategic plan and when capitation rates or other payment mechanisms are at an acceptable level. However, the HMO's ability to generate business for the hospital depends on its own financial strengths. The evaluation of an HMO includes looking at the sources of capital from which the HMO is financing its services; the reserve requirements of the state and the HMO's ability to meet them; and the HMO's long-term financial strength.

Rate Development and Premium Structure

Evaluating the capitation rates developed by the HMO for both physician and hospital services is paramount in determining the HMO's financial health and its suitability as a contracting partner. Hospitals need to understand how capitation rates are developed and what their impact may be on payment to the hospital and should develop a policy on whether or not to accept capitation arrangements. Rates may apply to different sets of benefits, they may or may not be adjusted for age and sex, and they can also involve varying degrees of protection against the cost of caring for catastrophically ill patients.

The issue of experience rating versus community rating is of great importance to hospitals contracting with HMOs. *Experience rating* takes into consideration the individual employer's claims experience for the previous year, whereas *community rating* bases rates on the aggregate claims experience of all employers contracting with an individual HMO. According to current HMO federal regulations HMOs must use the community-rating method, whereas CMPs may use the experience-rating approach. However, as a result of the development of the CMP program and other changes in the federal HMO act, HMOs are moving to experience-rated contracts.

The marketability and flexibility of experience-rated contracts should be evaluated, especially when capitation is being considered as the method of payment. Often, HMOs offer a hospital a capitation payment based on volume; if this is the case, the demographic mix of the HMO's members is important in evaluating the capitation payment because demographic mix relates to patient mix and consumption of services. Also, the benefits packages being offered by the HMO and the financial capacity of the hospital to provide the services called for should be closely examined.

If the hospital that serves large numbers of Medicare patients is considering CMP contracting, the hospital needs assurances that the offered payment amount, which may reflect the amount paid by HCFA to the CMP, can meet and cover the cost of the care the hospital is providing. Further, CMP payment amounts may possibly be reduced over time, reflecting the federal government's attempt to contain Medicare expenditures. Such actions may erode the profitability of the hospital-CMP arrangements.

Further, when evaluating the potential effectiveness of an HMO, the hospital should examine the HMO's premium structure and its competitiveness in the marketplace. The premium that an HMO offers to employers is a significant contributing factor in the employer's decision to offer the HMO to its employees. The premiums developed by the HMO are generally a combination of a price that is competitive with the employer's indemnity premium and the anticipated exposure of the group.

Payment Issues and Assumption of Risk

An HMO may use a number of different payment arrangements when contracting for services. Contracts between the HMO and the hospital can be as simple as an agreement to receive full charges or as complex as an arrangement in which an HMO contracts on a capitation basis (various payment options are shown in figures 2-2 and 2-3). Hospitals are frequently compensated by HMOs on a discount or per diem basis similar to arrangements found in PPO and direct employer contracting. The discussion in this section focuses on capitation because its use is growing and because it is found primarily in HMO contracting.

Capitation versus Fee for Service

Health maintenance organizations are moving toward capitation as a means of shifting risk to providers and improving the efficiencies of providing care to beneficiaries. As a practical matter, capitation arrangements are based on a payment per member of the plan per month; whereas fee-for-service payments, whether they are full charges, discounted charges, or per diem payments, are based on a per procedure basis or at least a per day basis.

From the HMO's perspective, fee-for-service payment systems are inefficient in two basic areas: billing and financial incentives. In fee-for-service payment arrangements, billing and associated claims processing are somewhat burdensome to both the hospital and the HMO, and as a result, more administrative resources are consumed than in capitation arrangements.

In a fee-for-service system, the HMO contracting providers lack financial incentives to provide health care service in a cost-effective manner. In a well-managed system, health problems receive cost-effective and high-quality treatment, and health promotion and preventive health care are emphasized. However, a fee-for-service system has no built-in rewards for providers to participate in these types of activities.

General Characteristics of Capitation Arrangements

Capitation payment systems can be structured in a number of ways, but the general characteristics of all systems are as follows:

- The provider receives a monthly payment on behalf of each enrollee. This payment does not vary according to the volume or intensity of services provided.
- The provider is required to deliver a specified range of services per member that corresponds to the monthly rate.
- When the costs of providing care to an enrollee exceed the capitation payment, the provider absorbs part, if not all, of the loss.
- When medical costs are, on average, held within the capitation payment, the provider keeps part, if not all, of the savings.

Some capitation arrangements also include profit-sharing arrangements between the hospital's contracting physicians and other providers involved in the HMO. Further, HMOs may negotiate favorable payment arrangements on a discount or full-charge basis for outpatient services or for such ancillary services as laboratory and pharmacy. When factored in with the capitation arrangement, this provision may also allow a profit margin for a hospital.

Stop-Loss Coverage

Capitation contracts frequently require a hospital to purchase some type of stop-loss coverage, sometimes called reinsurance coverage, to protect against catastrophic cases. Hospitals may be required to purchase coverage of anywhere from $25,000 to $150,000 per occurrence from the HMO itself or independently. These dollar amounts represent a provider's maximum liability under this arrangement. Once the hospital reaches the stop-loss coverage on either a specific or aggregate basis, the insurance carrier issuing the reinsurance policy assumes financial coverage. The lower the dollar amount of the stop-loss coverage purchased, the lower the hospital's risk, but lower stop-loss amounts carry higher premiums.

Advantages and Disadvantages of Capitation

The primary advantage of capitation is the financial reward for practicing cost-effective medicine. Other advantages are predictable cash flow and the elimination of the billing process and potential lengthy delays associated with claims payment. The primary disadvantage of capitation for the provider is that the provider assumes full risk: the provider must face the possibility that the treatment required by an HMO member will exceed the capitation amount. For some hospitals, this risk far outweighs the advantage of predictable cash flow and potential financial rewards.

A capitation system places virtually all of the responsibility and rewards for effective utilization management in the hands of the provider. Shouldering all the responsibility and getting all the rewards may or may not be to the advantage of a contracting hospital.

Organizational Structure

An HMO may be organized as a staff model, group model, network model, or individual practice association (IPA). The *staff model* delivers service through a group practice specifically established to provide medical services to this HMO's members; physicians are salaried staff of the HMO. The *group model* contracts with a group practice to provide medical services; the group is usually compensated on a capitation basis but may be compensated on a fee-for-service basis. Regardless of the type of group compensation, the individual physician's compensation is determined by the group itself. The *network model* contracts with two or more group practices to provide health care services. The *IPA model* is an association of physicians with varied specialties and in varied locations that generally provides health care services on a fee-for-service basis but may receive capitated payment.

In the case of group and staff models, hospital-HMO contracts may be between the HMO itself and the hospital. In an IPA-model

HMO, contracts may be between the hospital and an IPA or between the hospital and an HMO that is contracting with IPAs.

Hospitals contracting with a staff-model HMO may be subject to the most stringent utilization management controls. This type of model may be less marketable because the employee has fewer choices of hospitals and physicians that can provide them with health care.

At the other end of the spectrum is the IPA-model HMO. The IPA often offers employees the greatest number of physicians and hospitals from which to choose a health care provider, and so this model may have a marketing advantage. The IPA model may be the most difficult to control because the physicians are widely dispersed. Utilization management is often more difficult to control in the IPA HMO.

The group-model and network-model HMO fall somewhere between the staff and IPA models in regard to utilization control and marketability. The hospital must carefully weigh the differences in the various types of HMOs and assess the HMO's ability to attract employers as sponsors and employees as subscribers.

Political Issues

Hospitals contracting with HMOs may experience some political constraints relative to the size of the community in which they are operating, the number of contracts they already have with HMOs, and their past experiences in HMO contracting. Board members may not agree with the strategy of discounting price in exchange for the chance of increased patient days. However, HMO contracts may be less politically disturbing than other types of contracts discussed in previous chapters.

Political conflicts may arise when a hospital has sponsored its own HMO or is an equity owner in an HMO and is presented with the opportunity to contract with other HMOs. Contracting with other HMOs may reduce the marketability of the HMO with which the hospital is affiliated. However, seeking other HMO contracts may be in the best financial interests of the hospital.

Medical staffs that have had little experience with HMOs are likely to react negatively to the first HMO in their area. Generally, physicians are hesitant to participate in an HMO, but after they come to realize its potential market value, they may express a greater interest in joining. However, medical staffs with significant HMO experience may sometimes want to avoid further involvement. Also of concern to hospitals is how many members of the medical staff have joined HMOs and how this affiliation affects hospital admissions. The hospital should consider contracting with all the HMOs that a major portion of their medical staff affiliate with.

Another consideration is how many of the hospital's total and private-pay patient days the HMO represents. A potential to represent 30 percent to 50 percent of patient days gives the HMO considerable political power over the hospital. Some HMOs account for up to 70 percent or 80 percent of a hospital's patient days. In effect, such HMOs "control" the hospital and can make most policy decisions because of their purchasing power.

When evaluating an HMO arrangement, a hospital should also consider what other arrangements or contracts it is involved in and whether the HMO contract being considered has an exclusivity clause. Some HMOs do have exclusivity clauses in their legal contracts with hospitals and physicians. However, depending on the size of the community and the number of hospitals, exclusivity arrangements may not be marketable to hospitals, considering the possible negative competitive effect of such agreements.

Management Information Systems Requirements

In HMO contracting, as in all risk-taking situations, extensive tracking of utilization and cost issues is important to the hospital's and the HMO's financial strength. The hospital's responsibilities in collecting and analyzing this information should be carefully detailed within a contract.

A hospital contracting with an HMO should have a management information system (MIS) that can provide an intensive internal utilization review of HMO patients. This system should be able to sort and track patients by HMO and determine utilization patterns for each HMO group. Such data help both parties in renegotiating the contract based on experience. The data also help the hospital to determine if its current patient base is simply shifting to the HMO or if it is gaining additional market share by attracting new HMO patients. Hospitals should also profile the participating physicians to identify the overutilizers and underutilizers of patient days and resources. In many cases, continuing education may solve the problem of a physician who is abusive of the hospital's resources. In a capitation arrangement in which the hospital is assuming full financial risk, precise cost accounting and tracking systems for HMO patients are required. (Contract monitoring through system reports is described in chapter 1.)

Quality Assurance and Utilization Management Systems

Even though the chief concern of some HMOs in contracting with hospitals is price, most HMOs have developed criteria that take quality assurance and utilization management practices into consideration. A hospital's UR program may be carefully evaluated by an HMO that is considering a contracting arrangement with the hospital.

An HMO's internal utilization management and quality assurance system closely scrutinizes the number of patient days and the use of ancillary services at each hospital with which the HMO has a contract. The hospital must consider whether the utilization goals of an HMO are indeed appropriate and achievable and whether the hospital can reach these goals if achievement of these goals is the basis for payment. Further, from the hospital's perspective, any increase in operating costs resulting from the operation of this utilization management program should be evaluated in terms of its overall effectiveness and the financial feasibility of the contract.

A key issue for hospitals contracting with HMOs is answering the questions of who makes preadmission certification decisions, what are their qualifications, how smoothly does the process work, and what are the explicit requirements of the hospital in this process. In addition, because the goal of HMOs is to decrease inpatient utilization, the hospital should try to determine the HMO's ability to direct patients to outpatient and other hospital services as well as to attract more patients to the hospital's inpatient services.

Operational Issues

Once a hospital has signed an HMO contract, be it through an IPA structure or directly with a staff-model or group-model HMO, several operational issues should be discussed and monitored. These issues include data requirements, frequency of reporting the data, reporting format, payment of bills, member eligibility, and any specific utilization management activities that are delegated to the hospital.

Specific reporting formats and their applicability to a hospital's management information system should be discussed and negotiated. Further, the specific requirements of the utilization management system in terms of preadmission review, criteria for certification of patient admissions, concurrent and retrospective reviews, frequency of patient reviews, and specific billing procedures should be itemized in a contract.

Many HMOs monitor utilization management data, closely scrutinizing hospital utilization, and make relatively few demands on the hospital. However, in a capitation arrangement, more and more responsibility is delegated to the hospital.

The hospital's admissions procedures as they pertain to each contracting HMO should be fully spelled out in a hospital operating procedures manual. These procedures include types of employee identification for determining eligibility, level of benefits, and any other procedures required of a patient, such as obtaining a second opinion for surgical procedures, and procedures for gathering data and performing required utilization reviews.

Negotiations

As stated in chapter 5 on negotiating with PPOs, hospitals should develop a basic strategy for contracting with HMOs that may be one of the following:

- Contracting with all HMOs
- Contracting with a selected few, with definite criteria for selection
- Contracting with no HMOs

The appropriate strategy, as is the case with direct employer and PPO contracting, depends on the demographics of the marketplace and the hospital's strategic plan for establishing and maintaining long-term competitiveness.

A number of political issues based on the market power of the HMO arise when contracting with HMOs. An HMO that is able to deliver a sizable market share may dictate payment arrangements and administrative procedures that are more favorable to the HMO than to the hospital. The hospital needs to evaluate what it clearly gains from such an arrangement against its existing market alternatives.

Prior to negotiations, hospitals should evaluate the HMO organization itself. Matters to be examined include:

- Structure of the HMO (group, staff, network, or IPA)
- Short-term and long-term financial stability
- Management structure, governance structure, and tax status
- Reputation of the HMO for quality and service
- Utilization management program operated by the HMO and its effect on accessibility to care for members
- The HMO's information systems and its ability to share or desire to share information it gathers with the hospital
- Overall market share of the HMO within the community as well as its ability to build market share for the hospital, including evaluation of other hospitals under contract with the HMO and their competitiveness with the negotiating hospital
- Examination of any political reasons to contract or not to contract with an HMO, including religious mission or philosophy or other special issues

As hospitals are inundated with requests for contracts from several HMOs, PPOs, and other organizations, they must select those that will have some type of positive impact on the hospital. Getting to know the management and the operating systems of an HMO is important even in the initial stages of contract development.

The first thing a hospital should do when it receives an HMO contract proposal is to evaluate the offered rates in terms of payment methodology and level of risk. Health maintenance organizations have often contracted on per diem rates, either multiple or flat per diem, or on a discount-off-charges basis and are now moving to capitation arrangements. Hospitals must evaluate the short-term and long-term effects of these different payment arrangements on their internal cash flow. These payment arrangements can have an effect on the level of risk being acquired by the hospital and on the hospital's ability to cover cost and ensure a profit on that group of patients. Again, profitability is related to the age, sex, and geographic demographics of the HMO population. Often an actuarial study will have been completed by the HMO's actuaries, and a hospital should ask to review the study. Also, at the end of each contract year, a hospital should consider an actuarial evaluation of its own overall level of risk based on multiple risk-sharing contracts. Such a study is especially important if the hospital is operating under capitated or case rates.

Finally, the HMO contract, like the direct employer and PPO contracts, should be evaluated in terms of specific issues, including use of a hospital's name in marketing, termination provision applying to both parties, any volume guarantees or rate arrangements that are tied to a volume percentage, and UR requirements. Other issues of importance are the level of services being contracted for (specialty only, full-service, or extended vertically integrated services); the role of the physician organization; the responsibility for verification of eligibility of beneficiaries or members; administrative procedures such as billing, admissions, and payment time frames; and distribution of hospital-specific information. Further, confidentiality of patient data should also be covered within a contract.

Negotiation targets for the hospital should be to arrange for the most appropriate payment level and volume potential while maintaining a level of autonomy and agreement with the hospital's philosophy. The negotiation process requires evaluation of the contracting HMO and the contract and the acceptance or rejection of the offered arrangements. Many of the negotiating tips discussed in chapters 4 and 5 also apply to negotiation between hospitals and HMOs.

Conclusion

Hospitals are becoming increasingly selective in their contracting arrangements as they evaluate the ability of HMOs and other managed care programs to deliver patients. Understanding the marketplace and the HMO players within that marketplace, evaluating the financing and payment issues and organizational structures, being attentive to state and federal legal issues, and understanding the assumption of risk—all these issues are important for a contracting hospital to consider.

This chapter has focused on the process of contracting between hospitals and HMOs. An evaluation of the HMO's market position, financial goals, and potential benefit to the hospital is a key element in the process. Financial planning issues, marketing issues, and the benefits or problems related to capitated arrangements must be carefully considered in the contract negotiation process as must related political, organizational, and operational issues.

Key considerations in contracting with an HMO include the following:

- Often the hospital is placed in a reactive position, with less than optimal communication between the hospital and the HMO. Gathering maximum information from the HMO before making a decision is important.
- The hospital must evaluate the reputation and track record of the HMO to determine if it desires to have its name linked to the HMO, and the hospital must also try to determine the HMO's long-term financial and market viability.
- The hospital should carefully assess the level of risk it can assume. Actuarial analysis and an evaluation of service and demographic issues may be required.
- The hospital should determine the pros and cons of market-share exclusivity.